KETO DIET FOR WOMEN AFTER 50

How To Regain Your
Metabolism, Balance Hormones,
And Get Rid Of Belly Fat Quickly.
Including 91 Healthy, Simple
Recipes And A 30-Day Meal Plan

Gracelynn Rogers

Table of Contents

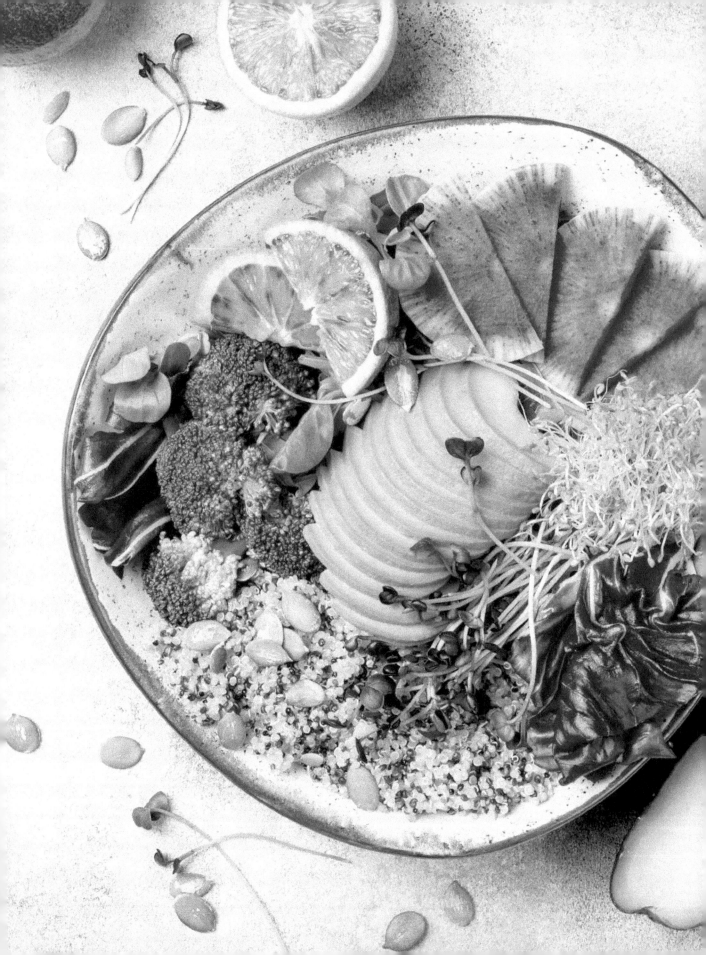

INTRODUCTION

What is a Keto Diet?

The name "Keto" comes from the word "ketogenic" which refers to the metabolic state of ketosis that starts in the body when carbohydrate intake is suddenly reduced and replaced with healthy fats. Most people start a ketogenic diet to lose weight, not just in water weight but in abdominal and other stored fat. It resembles the Atkins and other low-carb diets. The primary guideline is to drastically reduce your consumption of carbohydrates and replace them with healthy fats. This dramatic reduction in carbohydrates helps your body enter a metabolic state called ketosis in which your body burns fat for fuel rather than glucose.

The average person eats foods loaded in carbohydrates, the liver then converts glucose. Your body creates insulin in order to move the glucose into the bloodstream, which distributes it throughout your body and brain. The body's primary source of energy is glucose whenever carbohydrates are present in the body. Your body will always use glucose over fat or any other energy source.

The keto diet is focused on not using glucose as your energy source but instead fat. Once your body enters ketosis, your body becomes effective at burning fat, losing weight, and overall improving health. It also converts fat into ketones inside your liver, which can supply energy for the brain. The ketogenic diet can cause also cause a massive reduction in blood sugar and insulin levels.

The keto diet or the ketogenic diet requires you to follow a meal plan that is low in carbs and high in fat. It has some similarities with diet plans like the Atkin's diet and other low-carb meal plans. The goal of this diet is to increase the fat content in the body and reducing the carbohydrate content to push your body into the ketosis state which turns you into a fat burning machine.

There are several types of Ketogenic diet that you could adapt and maintain. These include;

The Standard Ketogenic Diet (SKD)

In simple terms, this is a very low-carb diet accompanied by high-fats and moderate protein that are consumed by human beings. It consists of 70% to 75% fats, 20% protein and about 5% to 10% carbs. This translates to about 20 – 45 grams of carbohydrates, 40 – 65 grams of proteins, but no set limits for fats, which makes up for large parts of the diet. This is because fats are what provide the calories which constitute energy and make the diet a successful Ketogenic diet. Additionally, there is no limit to the fats because different human beings have different energy requirements. The Standard Ketogenic Diet is successful in assisting people in losing weight, improving the body's glucose as well as improving heart health.

Targeted Ketogenic Diet (Tkd)

This type of Ketogenic Diet focuses its attention on the addition of carbs during workout sessions only. This type of Ketogenic diet is almost similar to the Standard Ketogenic Diet except for the fact that carbohydrates are all but consumed during workout sessions. This type of diet is solely based on the idea that the body will effectively and efficiently process carbohydrates consumed before or during a workout session. This is because the diet assumes that the muscles would be bound to demand more energy, which would be provided by the carbohydrates consumed and be processed quickly since the body is in an active state. This diet, in simpler terms, is a diet caught up between the Cyclical Ketogenic diet and the Standard Ketogenic Diet, which allows room for consumption of carbohydrates on the days that you would decide to work out only.

High-Protein Ketogenic Diet

This type of Ketogenic Diet advocates for more protein compared to the Standard Ketogenic Diet. This diet consists of 35% protein, 60% fats, and 5% carbs, unlike the Standard Ketogenic Diet. Research has dramatically suggested that this diet would be useful for you if you are attempting to lose weight. However, unlike other types of the Ketogenic diet, no research has been dedicated to showing if there are any side effects of adapting to the diet for elongated periods.

Recurring Ketogenic Diet (RKD)

This kind of Ketogenic Diet focuses on higher-carb re-feeds, for instance, 5 Ketogenic days and two high-carb days, and this cycle is repeated. This diet is also known as the carb backloading. It is often intended for athletes because the diet allows their bodies to recover the glycogen lost as a result of workouts or intense sporting activities.

Very Low Carbs Ketogenic Diet (VLCKD)

As stated prior, a Ketogenic diet will most likely consist of very low carbs; thus, this diet often refers to the characteristics of the Standard Ketogenic Diet.

The Well Formulated Ketogenic Diet

This term is a result of one of the leading researchers into the Ketogenic diet, Steve Phinney. As the name suggests, this diet has its fats, carbohydrates, and proteins well-formulated, that it meets the standards of a Ketogenic diet. This diet is also similar to the Standard Ketogenic Diet, and this means that it creates room for your body to undergo Ketosis effectively.

The Mct Ketogenic Diet

The diet is also related to the Standard Ketogenic Diet only that it derives most of its fats from medium-chain triglycerides (MCTs). This diet will often use coconut oil, which has high levels of MCTs. This diet has been reported to efficiently treat epilepsy because of its concept that MCTs give your body enough room to consume carbohydrates as well as proteins and still maintain your body's Ketosis. This is a result of MCTs providing more ketones per gram in fat, contrary to the long-chain triglycerides, which are more common in the average dietary fats. However, MCTs could lead to diarrhea as well as stomach upsets if this diet is consumed in large quantities on its own. To handle, it is wise to prepare a meal with a balance of both MCTs and fats with no MCTs. There is no evidence to prove that this diet could as well have benefits in your attempt to losing weight or if the diet could regulate your body's blood sugar.

The Calorie Restricted Ketogenic Diet

This is also related to the Standard Ketogenic Diet except that its calories are only limited to a given amount. Research has proven that Ketogenic diets could be successful whether the consumption of calories is restricted or not. The reason behind this is that the effect of consuming fats and your body being in Ketosis is a way in itself that prevents you from over-eating or eating beyond your limits.

There are numerous Ketogenic diets, but the Standard Ketogenic Diet and the High-Protein Ketogenic Diets are the most studied and most recommended for health issues. The Repeated (cyclical) and Targeted Ketogenic diets remain mostly practiced by athletes and bodybuilders and are more advanced than the Standard Ketogenic Diet and the High-Protein Ketogenic Diet. Visit and consult your local physician before opting to settle on any of the types of Ketogenic diets.

CHAPTER 1: BENEFITS OF KETO DIET FOR WOMEN OVER 50

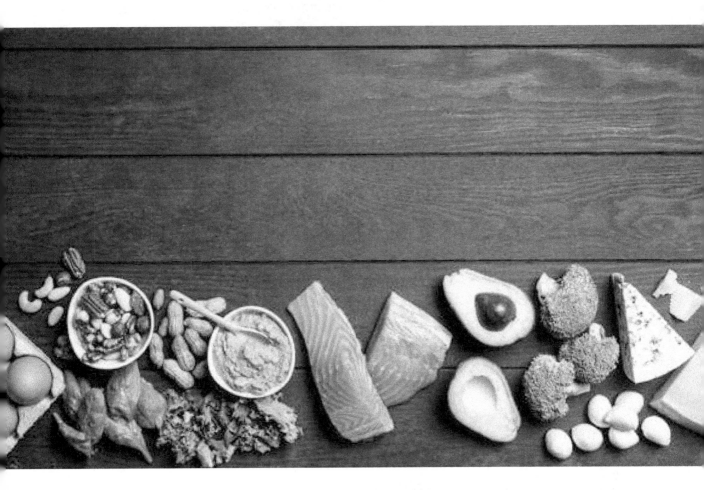

The Keto diet has become so popular in recent years because of the success people have noticed. Not only have they lost weight, but scientific studies show that the Keto diet can help you improve your health in many others. As when starting any new diet or exercise routine, there may seem to be some disadvantages, so we will go over those for the Keto diet. But most people agree that the benefits outweigh the change period!

Benefits/Advantages

Losing Weight

For most people, this is the foremost benefit of switching to Keto! Their previous diet method may have stalled for them, or they were noticing weight creeping back on. With Keto, studies have shown that people have been able to follow this diet and relay fewer hunger pangs and suppressed appetite while losing weight at the same time! You are minimizing your carbohydrate intake, which means more occasional blood sugar spikes. Often, those fluctuations in blood sugar levels make you feel hungrier and more prone to snacking in between meals. Instead, by guiding the body towards ketosis, you are eating a more fulfilling diet of fat and protein and harnessing energy from ketone molecules instead of glucose. Studies show that low-carb diets effectively reduce visceral fat (the fat you commonly see around the abdomen increases as you become obese). This reduces your risk of obesity and improves your health in the long run.

Reduce the Risk of Type 2 Diabetes

The problem with carbohydrates is how unstable they make blood sugar levels. This can be very dangerous for people who have diabetes or are pre-diabetic because of unbalanced blood sugar levels or family history. Keto is an excellent option because of the minimal intake of carbohydrates it requires. Instead, you are harnessing most of your calories from fat or protein, which will not cause blood sugar spikes and, ultimately, less pressured the pancreas to secrete insulin. Many studies have found that diabetes patients who followed the Keto diet lost more weight and eventually reduced their fasting glucose levels. This is monumental news for patients with unstable blood sugar levels or hopes to avoid or reduce their diabetes medication intake.

Improve Cardiovascular Risk Symptoms to Lower Your Chances of Having Heart Disease

Most people assume that following Keto that is so high in fat content has to increase your risk of coronary heart disease or heart attack. But the research proves otherwise! Research shows that switching to Keto can lower your blood pressure, increase your HDL good cholesterol, and reduce your triglyceride fatty acid levels. That's because the fat you are consuming on Keto is healthy and high-quality fats, so they reverse many unhealthy symptoms of heart disease. They boost your "good" HDL cholesterol numbers and decrease your "bad" LDL cholesterol numbers. It also reduces the level of triglyceride fatty acids in the bloodstream. A top-level of these can lead to stroke, heart attack, or premature death. And what are the top levels of fatty acids linked to?

High Consumption of Carbohydrates

With the Keto diet, you are drastically cutting your intake of carbohydrates to improve fatty acid levels and improve other risk factors. A 2018 study on the Keto diet found that it can improve 22 out of 26 risk factors for cardiovascular heart disease! These factors can be critical to some people, especially those who have a history of heart disease in their family.

Increases the Body's Energy Levels

Let's briefly compare the difference between the glucose molecules synthesized from a high carbohydrate intake versus ketones produced on the Keto diet. The liver makes ketones and use fat molecules you already stored. This makes them much more energy-rich and an endless source of fuel compared to glucose, a simple sugar molecule. These ketones can give you a burst of energy physically and mentally, allowing you to have greater focus, clarity, and attention to detail.

Decreases Inflammation in the Body

Inflammation on its own is a natural response by the body's immune system, but when it becomes uncontrollable, it can lead to an array of health problems, some severe and some minor. The health concerns include acne, autoimmune conditions, arthritis, psoriasis, irritable bowel syndrome, and even acne and eczema. Often, removing sugars and carbohydrates from your diet can help patients of these diseases avoid flare-ups - and the delightful news is Keto does just that! A 2008 research study found that Keto decreased a blood marker linked to high inflammation in the body by nearly 40%. This is glorious news for people who may suffer from inflammatory disease and want to change their diet to improve.

Increases Your Mental Functioning Level

As we elaborated earlier, the energy-rich ketones can boost the body's physical and mental levels of alertness. Research has shown that Keto is a much better energy source for the brain than simple sugar glucose molecules are. With nearly 75% of your diet coming from healthy fats, the brain's neural cells and mitochondria have a better source of energy to function at the highest level. Some studies have tested patients on the Keto diet and found they had higher cognitive functioning, better memory recall, and were less susceptible to memory loss. The Keto diet can even decrease the occurrence of migraines, which can be very detrimental to patients.

Decreases Risk of Diseases like Alzheimer's, Parkinson's, and Epilepsy

They created the Keto diet in the 1920s to combat epilepsy in children. From there, research has found that Keto can improve your cognitive functioning level and protect brain cells from injury or damage. This is very good to reduce the risk of neurodegenerative disease, which begins in the brain because of neural cells mutating and functioning with damaged parts or lower than peak optimal functioning. Studies have found that the following Keto can improve the mental functioning of patients who suffer from diseases like Alzheimer's or Parkinson's. These neurodegenerative diseases sadly have no cure, but the Keto diet could improve symptoms as they progress. Researchers believe that it's because cutting out carbs from your diet, which reduces the occurrence of blood sugar spikes that the body's neural cells have to keep adjusting to.

Keto Can Regulate Hormones in Women Who Have PCOS (Polycystic Ovary Syndrome) and PMS (Pre-Menstrual Syndrome)

Women who have PCOS suffer from infertility, which can be very heartbreaking for young couples trying to start a family. For this condition, there is no known cure, but we believe it's related to many similar diabetic symptoms like obesity and a high level of insulin. This causes the body to produce more sex hormones, which can lead to infertility. The Keto diet paved its way as a popular way to regulate insulin and hormone levels and increase a woman's chances of getting pregnant.

CHAPTER 2: IMPORTANCE OF LIFESTYLE

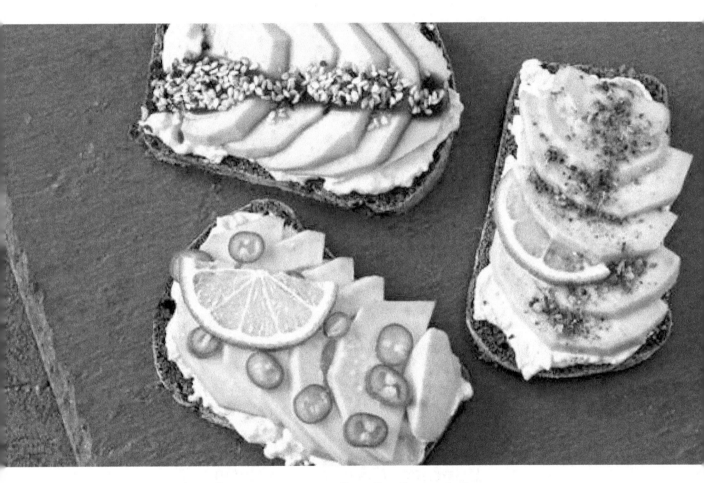

Enhance Your Physical Activity

Taking part in physical activity may support ketone fixations during carb restriction. This effect can be improved by working in a quick paced state.

Exercising

Exercising offers a plethora of benefits to all, regardless of your age! Healthy movement results in improved flexibility and more robust bones, which is quite essential for older folks. You see, as you age, your body's muscle mass starts to decrease. As we enter our fifties, adults begin to lose three to five percent of muscle mass as they enter each new decade.

However, we do realize how the thought of exercising regularly at an older age can seem like a challenge, especially if you're feeling let down with frequent aches and pains. But in many ways, the benefits of exercising outweigh the potential risks. Let's dive into why exercising is such important for seniors.

Benefits Exercising for Seniors

While you may be having thoughts about exercising, here are a couple of services that you can't ignore:

Prevents Diseases

Regular physical activity has been known to reduce the risks of diseases such as diabetes and heart disease. Mainly because exercise strengthens overall immune functioning, which is particularly beneficial for seniors who are often immunocompromised. Even if you can't hit the gym, some form of light exercise can play an integral role in disease management.

Helps Increase Social Ties and Prevents Isolation

Aging can be a daunting process, but it becomes fun when a community surrounds you. Opting for yoga or fitness classes not only makes exercising more fun, but it also helps you strengthen social ties with other older adults in your neighborhood. It can help ward off the occasional loneliness that one is likely to feel at old age. Plus, this will help you stay committed to your goals and lead a healthier lifestyle.

Improves Cognitive Function

Regular exercise can also improve fine motor skills that boost cognitive function. Several studies have shown how exercising can reduce the risk of dementia.

Tips & Tricks Exercises for Seniors

Here is a list of tips exercises that people in their fifties and beyond can enjoy:

Light Weight Training

You can start with a little weight training to retain bone density and build muscle mass. If you're more interested in doing home exercises than joining the gym, invest in 2-pound weights, perform arm raises, and shoulder presses.

Ideally, we recommend that you join a fitness center or gym where you can meet like-minded folks. You can also get yourself a personal trainer who can guide customized workouts for you. Either way, remember to take it slow at first as you don't want to exert yourself too much.

Walking

If lifting weights isn't for you, good old-fashioned walking should also work for you. Consider taking a nice walk around your neighborhood or go to a park nearby. You'll be able to make some friends and enjoy the weather while you're at it too.

In case you'd rather workout at home, strap on a pedometer, and get going around the house. You'll get more out of this workout if you move your arms and lift your knees as you take each step.

Aerobics

Joining an aerobics class can significantly help you keep your muscles healthy while maintaining mobility. It will not only improve balance but will reduce the risk of falls, thus drastically improving the overall quality of your life as you grow older.

Many studies have also indicated how aerobic exercises can protect memory and sharpen your mind and improving cognitive function among older adults. If you're not comfortable joining a class, you'll find plenty of videos online. Aerobic exercises have also been known to get the heart pumping, improving cardiovascular help.

Swimming

Do you find regular exercise too dull? Swimming is a fun, impact-free exercise that can get yours through the day. It's almost pain-free and won't trouble your aging joints. Swimming offers resistance training and will help you get back up to your feet again.

Here's how it works: the water offers gentle resistance while giving you a cardiovascular workout too. It also builds muscle capacity and helps you build strength again.

Yoga

What's no to love about yoga? It's relaxing, it's healthy, and you can enjoy it with a group. Yoga does an excellent job of improving flexibility in your joints. It allows seniors to remain limber and maintain their sense of balance. If you have trouble moving about or stretching, then you can try chair yoga.

Some classic yoga poses that you might want to try out include seated forward bend, downward facing dog, and warrior.

Squats

When you're working on an exercise program, you shouldn't skip the idea of strength training. Squats happen to be an excellent way to strengthen the muscles of your lower body. Doing squats is relatively easy, and you won't need any sort of equipment except for maybe a chair to support yourself. However, if you have trouble with balance, we suggest you skip this exercise and opt for something much more straightforward.

Sit-Ups

It strengthens your core muscles, improves back pain problems, and balance. Performing simple sit-ups should do the job. You should feel the sensation in your core muscles.

CHAPTER 3: WHAT FOODS CAN BE EATEN IN THE KETO DIET AND WHY

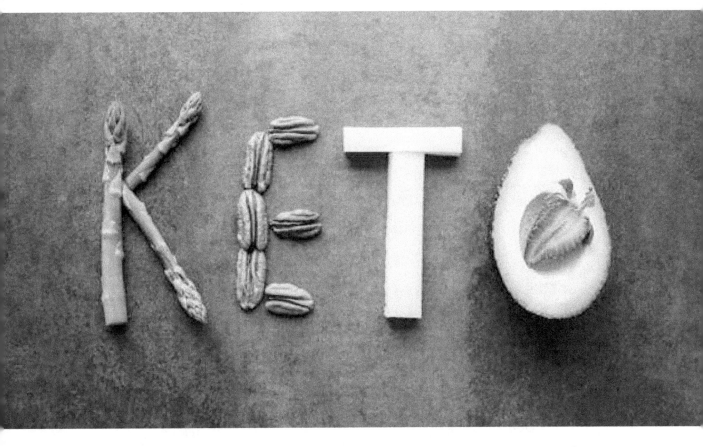

Now that we have gotten to the exciting part, it is time to learn what you can and cannot eat while following your new diet. Up until this point, you have most likely followed the food pyramid stating the importance of fruits and vegetables. While they are still going to be important for vitamins and nutrients, you are going to have to be selective. Below, you will find a complete list of foods you get to enjoy on the ketogenic diet!

Keto-Friendly Vegetables

Vegetables can be tricky when you are first starting the ketogenic diet. Some vegetables hold more carbohydrates than others. The simple rule that you need to remember is above the ground is good; below the ground is bad — got that?

Some popular above-ground vegetables you should consider for your diet (starting from the least carbs to the most carbs) include:

- Spinach
- Lettuce
- Avocado
- Asparagus
- Olives
- Cucumber
- Tomato
- Eggplant
- Cabbage
- Zucchini
- Cauliflower
- Kale
- Green Beans
- Broccoli
- Peppers
- Brussel Sprouts

And the below-ground vegetables you should avoid include:

- Carrots

- Onion

- Parsnip

- Beetroot

- Rutabaga

- Potato

- Sweet Potato

Every food that you put on your plate is comprised of three macronutrients: fat, protein, and carbohydrates. This will be an important lesson to learn before you begin your new diet, so be sure to take your time learning how to calculate them.

The golden rule is that meat and dairy are mostly made from protein and fat. Vegetables are mostly carbohydrates. Remember that while following the ketogenic diet, less than 5% of your calories need to come from carbohydrates. This is probably one of the trickiest tasks to get down when you are first getting started; there are hidden carbs everywhere! You will be amazed at how fast 20 g of carbs will go in a single day, much less a single meal!

When you are first getting started, you may want to dip your toes into the carb-cutting. As a rule, vegetables that have less than 5 net carbs can be eaten fairly freely. To make them a bit more ketogenic, I suggest putting butter on your vegetables to get a source of fat into your meal.

If you still struggle at the store, figuring out which vegetables are ketogenic, look for vegetables with leaves. Vegetables that have left are typically spinach and lettuce, both that are keto-friendly. Another rule to follow is to look for green vegetables. Generally, green vegetables like green bell peppers and green cabbage are going to be lower in carbs!

Keto-Friendly Fruits

Much like with the vegetables, some berries and fruits contain hidden carbs. As a general rule, the larger the amount of fruit, the more sugar it contains; this is why fruit is seen as nature's candy! On the ketogenic diet, that is a no go. While berries are going to be okay in moderation, the best is you leave the other fruits out for best results.

You may be thinking to yourself; I need to eat fruits for nutrients! The truth is, you can get the same nutrients from vegetables, costing you fewer carbohydrates on the ketogenic diet. While eating some berries every once in a while won't knock you out of ketosis, it is good to see how they affect you. But, if you feel like indulging in fruit as a treat, you can try some of the following:

- Raspberries
- Blackberries
- Strawberries
- Plum
- Kiwi
- Cherries
- Blueberries
- Clementine
- Cantaloupe
- Peach

Keto-Friendly Meat

On the ketogenic diet, meat is going to become a staple for you! When you are selecting your meats, try to stick with organic, grass-fed, and unprocessed. What I do want you to keep in mind is that the ketogenic diet is not meant to be high in protein, it is meant to be high in fat. People often link the ketogenic diet to a high meat diet, and that simply is not true. As you begin your diet, there is no need to have excess amounts of meat or protein. If you do have excess protein, it is going to be converted to glucose, knocking you right out of ketosis.

There are several different proteins that you will be able to enjoy while following the ketogenic diet. When it comes to beef, you will want to try your best to stick with the fattier cuts. Some of the better cuts would include ground beef, roast, veal, and steak. If poultry is more your style, look for the darker, fattier meats. Some good options for poultry selection would be wild game, turkey, duck, quail, and good old-fashioned chicken. Other options include:

- Pork Loin

- Tenderloin

- Pork Chops

- Ham

- Bacon

On your new diet, you will also be able to enjoy several different seafood dishes! At the store, you will want to look for wild-caught sources. Some of the better options include mahi-mahi, catfish, cod, halibut, trout, sardines, salmon, tuna, and mackerel. If shellfish is more your style, you get to enjoy lobster, muscles, crab, clams, and even oysters!

Keep in mind that when selecting your meats, try to avoid the cured and processed meats. These items, such as jerky, hot dogs, salami, and pepperoni, have many artificial ingredients, additives, and unnecessary sugars that will keep you from reaching ketosis. You know the better options now, stick with them!

Keto-Friendly Nuts

As you begin the ketogenic diet, there is a common misconception that you will now be able to eat as many nuts as you would like because they are high in fat. While you can enjoy a healthy serving of nuts, it is possible to go too nuts on nuts. Much like with the fruits and the vegetables, you would be surprised to learn that there are hidden carbohydrates here, too!

The lowest carb nuts you are going to find include macadamia nuts, brazil nuts, and pecans. These are fairly low in carbohydrates and can be enjoyed freely while following the ketogenic diet. These are all great options if you are looking for a healthy, ketogenic snack or something to toss in your salad.

When you are at the shop, you will want to avoid the nuts that have been treated with glazes and sugars. All of these extra add sugar and carbohydrates, which you are going to want to avoid. The higher carb nuts include cashews, pistachios, almonds, pine, and peanuts. These nuts can be enjoyed in moderation, but it would be better to avoid.

The issue with eating nuts is that it is easy to overindulge in them. While they are technically keto-friendly, they still contain a high number of calories. With that in mind, you should only be eating when you are hungry and need energy. On the ketogenic diet, you will want to avoid snacking between meals. You don't need the nuts, but they taste good! If you want to lose weight, put the nuts down, and stick to a healthier snack instead.

Keto-Friendly Snacks

On the topic of snacks, let's take a look at keto-friendly ones to have instead of a handful of nuts! Before we begin, keep in mind that if you are looking to lose weight, you will want to avoid snacking when possible. In the beginning, it may be tougher, but as you adapt to the keto diet, your meals should keep your hunger at bay for much longer.

If you are looking for something small to take the edge off your hunger pangs, look for easy whole foods, some of these basics would include eggs, cheese, cold cuts, avocados, and even olives. As long as you have these basics in your fridge, it should stop you from reaching for the high-carb foods.

If you are looking for a snack with more of a crunch, vegetable sticks are always a great option! There are plenty of dipping sauces to add fat to your meal, as well. On top of that, pork rinds are a delicious, zero-carb treat. Beef jerky is also a good option, as long as you are aware of how many carbohydrates are in a commercial package.

With the good options in mind, it's always good to take a look at the bad. When you are snacking, avoid the high-carb fruits, the coffee with creamer, and the sugar-juices. Before you started the ketogenic diet, these were probably the easy option. You'll also want to avoid the obvious candy, chips, and donuts. Just remember when you are selecting your foods, ask if it is fueling you or not.

Keto-Friendly Oils, Sauces, and Fats

On the ketogenic diet, the key to getting enough fat into your diet is going to depend on the sauces and oils you use with your cooking. When you put enough fat into your meals, this is what is going to keep you satisfied after every meal. The secret here is to be careful with the labels. You may be surprised to learn that some of your favorite condiments may have hidden sugars (looking at you, ketchup).

While you are going to have to be a bit more careful about your condiments, you can never go wrong with butter! Up until this point, you have probably been encouraged to consume a low-fat diet. Now, I want you to embrace the fat! You can put butter in absolutely anything! Put butter on your vegetables, stick it in your coffee and get creative!

Oils, on the other hand, can be a bit more complicated. You see, natural oils such as fish oil, sesame oil, almond oil, ghee, pure olive oil, and even peanut oil can be used on absolutely anything. What you want to avoid are the oils that have been created in the past sixty years or so. The oils you'll want to avoid include soy oil, corn oil, sunflower oil, and any vegetable oil. Unfortunately, these oils have been highly processed and may hinder your process.

Stick with these for your diet instead:

- Butter

- Vinaigrette

- Coconut Oil

- Mayo

- Mustard

- Guacamole

- Heavy Cream

- Thousand Island Dressing

- Salsa

- Blue Cheese Dressing

- Ranch Dip

- Pesto

When it comes to dairy, high fat is going to be your best option. Cheese and butter are great options but keep the yogurts in moderation. When it comes to milk, you will want to avoid that as there is extra sugar in milk. If you enjoy heavy cream, this can be excellent for your cooking but should be used sparingly in your coffee.

Keto-Friendly Beverages

Remember that staying hydrated, especially when you are first starting your new diet, is going to be vital! Your safest bet is to always stick with water. Whether you like your water sparkling or flat, this is always going to be a zero-carb option. If you are struggling with a headache or the keto fly, remember that you can always throw a dash of salt in there.

CHAPTER 4: WHAT FOODS TO AVOID IN THE KETO DIET AND WHY?

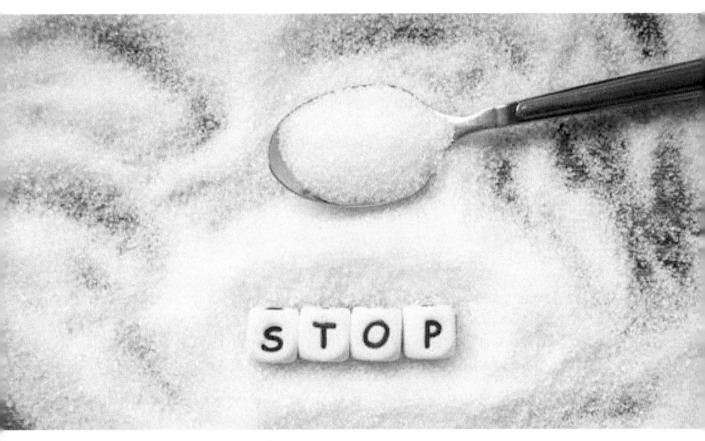

Because the diet is a keto, that means you need to avoid high-carbs food. Some of the food you avoid is even healthy, but it just contains too many carbs. Here is a list of typical food you should limit or avoid altogether.

Bread and Grains

No matter what form bread takes, they still pack a lot of carbs. The same applies to whole-grain as well because they are made from refined flour. So, if you want to eat bread, it is best to make keto variants at home instead.

Grains such as rice, wheat, and oats pack a lot of carbs as well. So, limit or avoid that as well.

Fruits

Fruits are healthy for you. The problem is that some of those foods pack quite a lot of carbs such as banana, raisins, dates, mango, and pear. As a general rule, avoid sweet and dried fruits.

Vegetables

Vegetables are just as healthy for your body. For one, they make you feel full for longer, so they help suppress your appetite. But that also means you need to avoid or limit vegetables that are high in starch because they have more carbs than fiber. That includes corn, potato, sweet potato, and beets.

Pasta

As with any other convenient food, pasta is rich in carbs. So, spaghetti or any different types of pasta are not recommended when you are on your keto diet.

Cereal

Cereal is also a considerable offender because sugary breakfast cereals pack a lot of carbs. That also applies to "healthy cereals." Just because they use other words to describe their product does not mean that you should believe them. That also applies to oatmeal, whole-grain cereals, etc.

Beer

In reality, you can drink most alcoholic beverages in moderation without fear. Beer is an exception to this rule because it packs a lot of carbs. Carbs in beers or other liquid are considered liquid carbs, and they are even more dangerous than substantial carbs.

Sweetened Yogurt

Yogurt is very healthy because it is tasty and does not have that many carbs. The problem comes when you consume yogurt variants rich in carbs such as fruit-flavored, low-fat, sweetened, or nonfat yogurt. A single serving of sweetened yogurt contains as many carbs as a single serving of dessert.

Juice

Fruit juices are perhaps the worst beverage you can put into your system when you are on a keto diet. Another problem is that the brain does not process liquid carbs the same way as stable carbs. Substantial carbs can help suppress appetite, but liquid carbs will only put your need into overdrive.

Low-fat and fat-free salad dressings

If you have to buy salads, keep in mind that commercial sauces pack more carbs than you think, especially the fat-free and low-fat variants.

Beans and Legumes

These are also very nutritious as they are rich in fiber. However, they are also rich in carbs. You may enjoy a small amount of them when you are on your keto diet, but don't exceed your carb limit.

Sugar

We mean sugar in any form, including honey. Foods that contain lots of sugar, such as cookies, candies, and cake, are forbidden on a keto diet or any other form of diet that is designed to lose weight. When you are on a keto diet, you need to keep in mind that your diet consists of food that is rich in fiber and nutritious. So, sugar is out of the question.

Chips and Crackers

These two are some of the most popular snacks. Some people did not realize that one packet of chips contains several servings and should not be all eaten in one go. The carbs can add up very quickly if you do not watch what you eat.

Milk

Milk also contains a lot of carbs on its own. Therefore, avoid it if you can even though milk is a good source of many nutrients such as calcium, potassium, and other B vitamins.

Gluten-Free Baked Goods

Gluten-free diets are trendy nowadays, but what many people don't seem to realize is that they pack quite a lot of carbs. That includes gluten-free bread, muffins, and other baked products. In reality, they contain even more carbs than their glutinous variant.

CHAPTER 5: DOES KETO DIET HAVE SIDE EFFECTS?

It would be very irresponsible of me if I only tell you all the good things about the Ketogenic Diet and ignore the side effects. The truth is that there are negative effects that could happen once you start the Ketogenic Diet – but that's actually true for all of them! All types of diet have negative effects to start with because your body has gotten used to bad habits. Once you make the shift to a more positive way of eating, the body sort of goes on a rebellious phase so it feels like everything is going wrong. For example, a person who used to eat lots of sugar in a day can have severe headaches once they start to avoid sugar. This is a withdrawal symptom and tells you that your diet is actually making positive changes to the body – albeit it takes a little bit of pain on your part.

So what can one expect when they make that change towards a healthy Ketogenic Diet? Here are some of the things to expect and of course – how to troubleshoot these problems.

Keto Breath

One of the most common side effects of a keto diet is bad breath. Not everyone who adopts the keto diet experiences this problem, but it is common. Bad breath comes as a result of internal metabolism processes. Your liver metabolizes the massive amounts of fat you are consuming and then converts them to ketone bodies such as acetone. These ketone bodies are broken down into smaller organizations and are then circulated inside your body. As the ketone bodies circulate, it gets into your lungs through the diffusion process, and eventually, it is exerted out through your breath.

How to Overcome Keto Breath?

You can control bad keto breath by increasing water intake. You can also get rid of this problem by practicing good oral hygiene like regularly brushing your teeth. Alternatively, you can mask ketosis odor using mints and gums. It is also advisable to eat slightly more carbs and less protein if you have this problem.

Keto Flu

You may experience symptoms resembling those of flu, especially during your first days on a keto diet. Such symptoms include aches, fatigue, cramping, skin rash, and diarrhea. The side effects are caused by dehydration as a result of your body losing a lot of water and electrolytes.

When your body uses fat to fuel its functions instead of using protein, you tend to lose more water and electrolytes through urination. The loss of water and electrolytes is accelerated further by the low insulin levels and muscle glycogen that accompanies the keto diet.

Besides, most keto diets consist of food with little water and potassium levels, further accelerating the loss of body water and electrolytes.

How to Overcome Keto Flu?

You can handle keto flu by drinking much water. You can also eat lots of soup. If you get enough rest, you will give your body enough energy to fight the flu on its own.

You need to lower the effects of keto flu by getting enough sleep. You can also drink much water to minimize the impact of keto flu. There are also some supplements found in natural sources like organic coffee or matcha tea that could help you overcome the flu. Make a point to get enough salts and electrolytes, too.

Fatigue

You may experience extreme feelings of tiredness once you adopt a keto diet. Fatigue is caused by a lack of glucose reaching your brain. Although this side effect will last for a few days, it could still cause much discomfort and worry on your part.

How to Overcome Keto Fatigue?

Drink much water and get enough rest. You can also avoid engaging in strenuous exercises. You can also eat healthy carbs to give you the extra energy your body needs.

GI Side Effects

Keto diet can also harm your digestive system over the long term. Keto diet has been thought to cause some stomach problems such as constipation high cholesterol levels, diarrhea, kidneys stones, and vomiting.

You may also experience abnormal stomach gas due to the sugar alcohols found in some keto diets, for example, the sugars found in some processed foods. The higher the amount of food you eat, the higher the impact of the side effects on you.

How to Control GI Problems When You Are on a Keto Diet?

Drink lots of water and eat high fiber foods such as fruits and vegetables to encourage the growth of beneficial bacteria in your GI system. Make it a habit of exercising regularly.

Weakened Immune System

Keto diets can also weaken the immune systems of some people. Studies suggest that keto foods could cause a condition called dysbiosis. Dysbiosis occurs when the balance of helpful and harmful bacteria is altered in your GI tract. The disruption is caused by the consumption of highly saturated fats and low fiber levels in your digestive system.

When you ingest diets with little prebiotic fiber, the number of beneficial bacteria decreases substantially in your digestive system. Your GI tract is the backbone of your immune system, and any compromise to it could have a negative impact on the immune functions leading to exposure to chronic diseases.

How to Avoid Weakened Immune System When on a Keto Diet?

Incorporate workouts to your keto diet. You can also eat high fiber food, such as fruits and vegetables. Also, ensure you drink lots of water.

Vitamin and Other Mineral Deficiencies

If you are on the keto diet, you may not receive enough vitamins and minerals needed for your body to function normally. Plant-based minerals such as calcium and vitamin D may not be present in your keto diet in the quantities required by your body. If these minerals decrease in your body for long periods, you may stand a high risk of getting lifestyle diseases such as heart failure.

Heart failure comes as a result of the hardening of your heart muscles because of the lack of enough selenium. Selenium is an essential immune-boosting antioxidant usually occurring in plant-based food. Lack of this critical antioxidant causes the hardening of your heart muscles leading to heart failure.

How to Treat the Deficiencies When You Are on a Keto Diet?

Eat lots of fruits and vegetables to get vitamins. You can also use beneficial supplements to treat any deficiencies, which comes with the keto diet.

Increased Risk of Chronic Disease

The Keto diet requires you to put a limit on the number of carbohydrates and protein you consume. When you eat much fat to get enough calories needed by your body, you will be limiting fiber-rich foods such as vegetables, fruits, or legumes. These foods are some of the best sources of immune-boosting nutrients needs by your body to stay healthy. Therefore, when you limit these nutrients in your body, you increase your risk of getting chronic diseases such as diabetes, cancer, high blood pressure.

Studies show that diets that are high in fruits and vegetables can significantly reduce chronic diseases. The more you consume them, the better you are health-wise. When you restrict their consumption, you tend to decrease their beneficial impacts.

How to Reduce the Risk of Chronic Diseases When on Keto Diets?

We'll say it again: drink lots of water. Eat lots of fruits and vegetables. You can also incorporate exercise into your keto diet to get the best results.

Chronic Inflammation

Studies show that when you consume high fats needed for Ketosis, your cholesterol and lipoprotein structure could be significantly altered and will result in inflammation over a while. Inflammation occurs when the cells of your body use much energy to accomplish their normal functioning. Chronic inflammation is also one of the causes of heart diseases.

How to Minimize Chronic Inflammation When on Keto Diets?

You can control the problem of inflammation by eating solid fats and oils. Ensure you also include high fiber foods in your daily intake, like fruits and vegetables.

The Challenge of Weight Cycling

When you restrict your eating diets for an extended period, you may end up gaining too much weight when not dieting, which you then go ahead and lose when on a diet. This process of alternating between weight gain and weight loss is what is referred to as weight cycling. Weight cycling can increase the risk of getting chronic diseases.

How to Control Weight Cycling?

You can control weight cycling by shortening the intervals between dieting and the days you are on free diets. You should gradually increase the amount of food you consume during your free diet days so that your body can have enough time to adjust to the changes in your program.

CHAPTER 6: BREAKFAST RECIPES

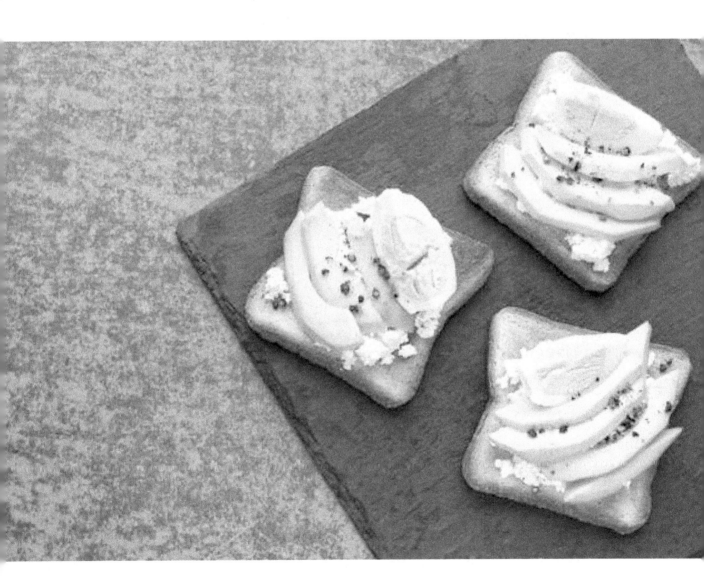

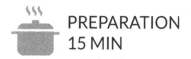
PREPARATION
15 MIN

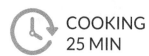
COOKING
25 MIN

SERVES
4

1. YOGURT WAFFLES

INGREDIENTS

- ½ cup golden flax seeds meal
- ½ cup plus 3 tablespoons almond flour
- 1-1½ tablespoons granulated erythritol
- 1 tablespoon unsweetened vanilla whey protein powder
- ½ teaspoon organic powder
- ¼ teaspoon xanthan gum
- Salt, as required
- 1 large organic egg, white and yolk separated

- 1 organic whole egg
- 2 tablespoons unsweetened almond milk
- 1½ tablespoons unsalted butter
- 3 ounces plain Greek yogurt
- ¼ teaspoon baking soda

DIRECTIONS

Preheat the waffle iron and then grease it

In a large bowl, add the flour, erythritol, protein powder, baking soda, baking powder, xanthan gum, salt, and mix until well combined

In a second small bowl, add the egg white and beat until stiff peaks form

In a third bowl, add 2 egg yolks, whole egg, almond milk, butter, yogurt and beat until well combined

Place egg mixture into the bowl of flour mixture and mix until well combined

Gently, fold in the beaten egg whites

Place ¼ cup of the mixture into preheated waffle iron and cook for about

4–5 minutes or until golden-brown

Repeat with the remaining mixture

Serve warm

Nutrition: Calories: 250 kcal Net Carbs: 3.2 g Total Carbs: 8.8 g Fiber: 5.6 g Sugar: 1.3 g Protein 8.4 g

2. BROCCOLI MUFFINS

PREPARATION
15 MIN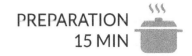

COOKING
20 MIN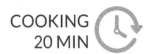

SERVES
5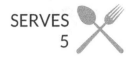

INGREDIENTS

- 2 tablespoons unsalted butter
- 6 large organic eggs
- ½ cup heavy whipping cream
- ½ cup Parmesan cheese, grated
- Salt and ground black pepper, as required
- 1¼ cup broccoli, chopped
- 2 tablespoons fresh parsley, chopped
- ½ cup Swiss cheese, grated

DIRECTIONS

Preheat your oven to 350 °F

Grease a 12-cup muffin tin

In a bowl, add the eggs, cream, Parmesan cheese, salt, black pepper and beat until well combined

Divide the broccoli and parsley in the bottom of each prepared muffin cup evenly

Top with the egg mixture, followed by the Swiss cheese

Bake for about 20 minutes, rotating the pan once halfway through

Remove from the oven and place onto a wire rack for about 5 minutes before serving

Carefully, invert the muffins onto a serving platter and serve warm

Nutrition: Calories: 231 kcal Net Carbs: 2 g Total Carbs: 2.5 g Fiber: 0.5 g Sugar: 0.9 g Protein: 13.5 g

PREPARATION
15 MIN

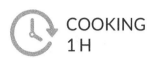

COOKING
1 H

SERVES
5

3. PUMPKIN BREAD

INGREDIENTS

- 1 2/3 cup almond flour
- 1½ teaspoons organic baking powder
- ½ teaspoon pumpkin pie spice
- ½ teaspoon ground cinnamon
- ½ teaspoon ground cloves
- ½ teaspoon salt
- 8 ounces cream cheese, softened
- 6 organic eggs, divided
- 1 tablespoon coconut flour
- 1 cup powdered erythritol, divided

- 1 teaspoon stevia powder, divided
- 1 teaspoon organic lemon extract
- 1 cup homemade pumpkin puree
- ½ cup coconut oil, melted

DIRECTIONS

Preheat your oven to 325 °F

Lightly, grease 2 bread loaf pans

In a bowl, place almond flour, baking powder, spices, salt and mix until well combined

In a second bowl, add the cream cheese, 1 egg, coconut flour, ¼ cup of erythritol, ¼ teaspoon of the stevia and with a wire whisk, beat until smooth

In a third bowl, add the pumpkin puree, oil, 5 eggs, ¾ cup of the erythritol, ¾ teaspoon of the stevia, and with a wire whisk, beat until well combined

Add the pumpkin mixture into the bowl of the flour mixture and mix until just combined

Place about ¼ of the pumpkin mixture into each loaf pan evenly

Top each pan with the cream cheese mixture evenly, followed by the remaining pumpkin mixture

Bake for about 50–60 minutes or until a toothpick inserted in the center comes out clean

Remove the bread pans from oven and place onto a wire rack and let it be for 10 minutes

With a sharp knife, cut each bread loaf in the desired-sized slices and serve

Nutrition: Calories: 216 kcal Net Carbs: 2.5 g Total Carbs: 4.5 g Fiber: 2 g Sugar: 1.1 g Protein: 3.4 g

4. SPINACH ARTICHOKE BREAKFAST BAKE

PREPARATION
15 MIN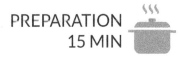

COOKING
20 MIN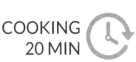

SERVES
7

INGREDIENTS

- ¼ c milk, fat-free
- ¼ tsp ground pepper
- 1/3 c red pepper, diced
- ½ c feta cheese crumbles
- ½ c scallions, finely sliced
- ¾ c canned artichokes, chopped, drained, & patted dry
- 1 ¼ tsp kosher salt
- 1 clove garlic, minced
- 1 tbsp dill, chopped

- 10 oz spinach, frozen, chopped & drained
- 2 tbsp parmesan cheese, grated
- 4 lg egg whites
- 8 lg eggs

DIRECTIONS

Preheat the oven to 375 °F and grease a large baking dish with nonstick spray or preferred fat source

In a small bowl, combine the spinach, artichoke, scallions, garlic, red pepper, and fill.

Combine completely and then pour into the baking dish, spreading into an even layer

In a mixing bowl, combine eggs, egg whites, salt, pepper, parmesan, and milk

Whisk until completely combined, then add feta and mix once more

Pour the egg mixture evenly over the vegetables in the baking dish

Bake for about 35 minutes, until a butter knife inserted in the center comes out clean

Allow to cool for about 10 minutes before cutting into eight equal pieces

Serve warm!

Nutrition: Calories: 574 kcal Carbohydrates: 2 g Protein: 47 g Fat: 54 g Sugar: 0.1 g Sodium: 254 mg Fiber: 0.7 g

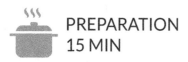

PREPARATION
15 MIN

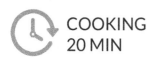

COOKING
20 MIN

SERVES
6

5. GRANOLA BARS

INGREDIENTS

- ► 2 c almonds, chopped
- ► ½ c pumpkin seeds, raw
- ► 1/3 c coconut flakes, unsweetened
- ► 2 tbsp hemp seeds
- ► ¼ c clear Sukrin Fiber Syrup
- ► ¼ c almond butter
- ► ¼ c erythritol, powdered, or equal measure of preferred sweetener
- ► 2 tsp vanilla extract
- ► 1/2 tsp sea salt

DIRECTIONS

Line a small, square baking dish with parchment paper

In a mixing bowl, combine almonds, pumpkin seeds, coconut flakes, and hemp seeds. Stir until evenly mixed

Over medium heat, combine the syrup, almond butter, sweetener, salt, and stir until it's smooth and easy to pull the spoon through

Remove the pan from the heat and stir the vanilla extract into the mixture

Pour the syrup over the seeds and stir completely

Pour the mixture into the baking dish and press evenly into one layer and press until the top is even

Let cool completely and slice into 12 bars

Nutrition: Calories: 254 kcal Carbohydrates: 2 g Protein: 42.5 g Fat: 47 g Sugar: 0.1 g Sodium: 145 mg Fiber: 0.7 g

6. GINGER FRENCH TOAST

PREPARATION
5 MIN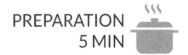

COOKING
10 MIN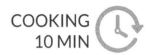

SERVES
2

INGREDIENTS

- ▶ 4 whole-wheat bread slices
- ▶ ½ cup low-fat milk
- ▶ 2 eggs, whisked
- ▶ 1 teaspoon ground ginger
- ▶ Cooking spray

DIRECTIONS

Spray the skillet with cooking spray

In the mixing bowl mix up milk and eggs

Then add ginger and dip the bread in the liquid

Roast the bread in the preheated skillet for 2 minutes from each side

Nutrition: Calories: 229 kcal Carbohydrates: 8 g Protein: 29.4 g Fat: 8 g Sugar: 2 g Sodium: 388 mg Fiber: 4 g

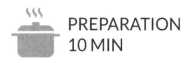
PREPARATION
10 MIN

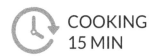
COOKING
15 MIN

SERVES
6

7. BAGELS WITH CHEESE

INGREDIENTS

▸ 2.5 cup mozzarella cheese
▸ 1 tsp baking powder
▸ 3 oz cream cheese
▸ 1.5 cup almond flour
▸ 2 eggs

DIRECTIONS

Shred the mozzarella and combine with the flour, baking powder, and cream cheese in a mixing container

Pop into the microwave for about one minute. Mix well

Let the mixture cool and add the eggs

Break apart into six sections and shape into round bagels

Note: You can also sprinkle with a seasoning of your choice or pinch of salt if desired

Bake them for approximately 12 to 15 minutes. Serve or cool and store

Nutrition: Net Carbohydrates: 8 g Protein: 19 g Total Fats: 31 g Calories: 374 kcal

8. BAKED APPLES

PREPARATION
10 MIN
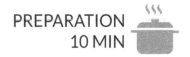

COOKING
1 H
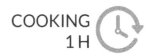

SERVES
4
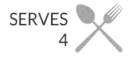

INGREDIENTS

- 4 tsp or to taste Keto-friendly sweetener
- 0.75 tsp cinnamon
- 0.25 cup chopped pecans
- 4 large granny Smith apples

DIRECTIONS

Set the oven temperature at 375 °F. Mix the sweetener with the cinnamon and pecans

Core the apple and add the prepared stuffing

Add enough water into the baking dish to cover the bottom of the apple

Bake them for about 45 minutes to 1 hour

Nutrition: Net Carbohydrates: 16 g Protein: 6.8 g Total Fats: 19.9 g Calories: 175 kcal

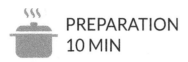

PREPARATION
10 MIN

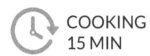

COOKING
15 MIN

SERVES
4

9. OMELET WITH PEPPERS

INGREDIENTS

- ► 4 eggs, beaten
- ► 1 tablespoon margarine
- ► 1 cup bell peppers, chopped
- ► 2 oz scallions, chopped

DIRECTIONS

Toss the margarine in the skillet and melt it

In the mixing bowl mix up eggs and bell peppers

Add scallions

Pour the egg mixture in the hot skillet and roast the omelet for 12 minutes

Nutrition: Calories: 102 kcal Carbohydrates: 7.3 g Protein: 6.1 g Fat: 10.8 g Sugar: 3 g Sodium: 98 mg Fiber: 0.8 g

10. AVOCADO EGG BOWLS

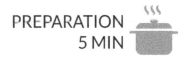

PREPARATION
5 MIN

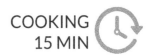

COOKING
15 MIN

SERVES
4

INGREDIENTS

- ▶ 1 avocado halved with the removed stone
- ▶ 1 tablespoon of salted butter
- ▶ 3 free-range eggs
- ▶ 3 rashers of bacon into little pieces
- ▶ black pepper and pinch of salt

DIRECTIONS

Begin by removing most of the avocado flesh, remaining just ½ inch on the avocado.

Put in butter into a large saucepan while it's heating. Let the butter melt in the pan. Crack the eggs and beat them in a jug, adding a little pepper and salt.

Put the bacon on one side of the pan and leave everything to fry for some minutes. Next, add the eggs to the opposite bottom of the pan and continue to stir until it is scrambled. The bacon and the eggs should be ready soon enough in 5 minutes. In case the scrambled eggs are done before the bacon, take it from the pan into a bowl.

Mix the pieces of the bacon and the scrambled eggs in the pot and add into the avocado bowls.

Nutrition: Calories: 500 Cal Fat: 26 g Carbs: 6 g Protein: 9 g Fiber: 9 g

CHAPTER 7: LUNCH RECIPES

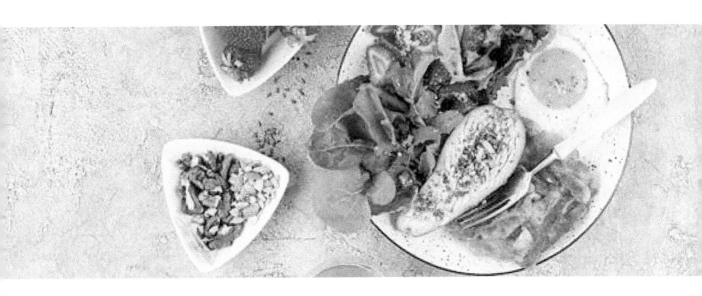

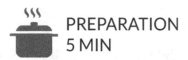

PREPARATION
5 MIN

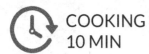

COOKING
10 MIN

SERVES
4

11. MUSHROOM & CAULIFLOWER RISOTTO

INGREDIENTS

▸ 1 grated head of cauliflower
▸ 1 cup vegetable stock
▸ 9 oz chopped mushrooms
▸ 2 tbsp butter
▸ 1 cup coconut cream

· ·

DIRECTIONS

Pour the stock in a saucepan. Boil and set aside

Prepare a skillet with butter and saute the mushrooms until golden

Grate and stir in the cauliflower and stock

Simmer and add the cream, cooking until the cauliflower is al dente

Serve

Nutrition: Net Carbohydrates: 4 g Protein: 1 g Total Fats: 17 g Calories: 186 kcal

12. PITA PIZZA

PREPARATION
15 MIN
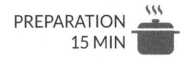

COOKING
10 MIN
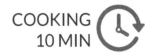

SERVES
2
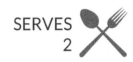

INGREDIENTS

- 0.5 cup marinara sauce
- 1 low-carb pita
- 2 oz cheddar cheese
- 14 slices pepperoni
- 1 oz roasted red peppers

DIRECTIONS

Program the oven temperature setting to 450 °F

Slice the pita in half and place onto a foil-lined baking tray

Rub with a bit of oil and toast for one to two minutes

Pour the sauce over the bread

Sprinkle using the cheese and other toppings

Bake until the cheese melts (5 min.)

Cool thoroughly

Nutrition: Net Carbohydrates: 4 g Protein: 13 g Total Fats: 19 g Calories: 250 kcal

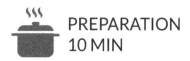
PREPARATION
10 MIN

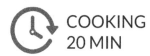
COOKING
20 MIN

SERVES
4

13. ITALIAN STYLE HALIBUT PACKETS

INGREDIENTS

- 2 cups cauliflower florets
- 1 cup roasted red pepper strips
- 1/2 cup sliced sun-dried tomatoes
- 4 (4-ounce) halibut fillets
- 1/4 cup chopped fresh basil
- Juice of 1 lemon
- 1/4 cup good-quality olive oil
- Sea salt, for seasoning
- Freshly ground black pepper, for seasoning

DIRECTIONS

Preheat the oven. Set the oven temperature to 400°F.

Make the packets.

Divide the cauliflower, red pepper strips, and sun-dried tomato between the four pieces of foil, placing the vegetables in the middle of each piece.

Top each pile with one halibut fillet, and top each fillet with equal amounts of the basil, lemon juice, and olive oil.

Fold and crimp the foil to form sealed packets of fish and vegetables and place them on the baking sheet.

Bake. Bake the packets for about 20 minutes, until the fish flakes with a fork.

Be careful of the steam when you open the packet!

Serve. Transfer the vegetables and halibut to four plates, season with salt and pepper, and serve immediately.

Nutrition: Calories: 313 Fat: 14.1g Fiber: 10.4g Carbohydrates:3.2 g Protein: 15.4g

14. TACO CASSEROLE

PREPARATION
10 MIN
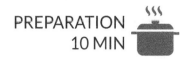

COOKING
20 MIN
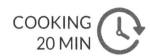

SERVES
8
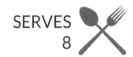

INGREDIENTS

- 1.5 to 2 lb ground turkey or beef
- 2 tbsp taco seasoning
- 8 oz shredded cheddar cheese
- 1 cup salsa
- 16 oz cottage cheese

DIRECTIONS

Heat the oven to reach 400 °F.

Combine the taco seasoning and ground meat in a casserole dish.

Bake it for 20 minutes.

Combine the salsa and both kinds of cheese. Set aside for now.

Carefully transfer the casserole dish from the oven.

Drain away the cooking juices from the meat.

Break the meat into small pieces and mash with a masher or fork.

Sprinkle with cheese.

Bake in the oven for 15 to 20 more minutes until the top is browned.

Nutrition: Net Carbohydrates: 6 g Protein: 45 g Total Fats: 18 g Calories: 367 kcal

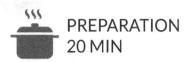 **PREPARATION**
20 MIN

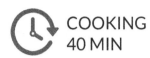 **COOKING**
40 MIN

 **SERVES**
4

15. BEEF WELLINGTON

INGREDIENTS

- ► 2 (4-ounce) grass-fed beef tenderloin steaks, halved
- ► Salt and ground black pepper, as required
- ► 1 tablespoon butter
- ► 1 cup mozzarella cheese, shredded
- ► 1/2 cup almond flour
- ► 4 tablespoons liver pate

DIRECTIONS

Preheat your oven to 400°F.

Grease a baking sheet.

Season the steaks with pepper and salt.

Sear the beef steaks for about 2–3 minutes per side.

In a microwave-safe bowl, add the mozzarella cheese and microwave for about 1 minute.

Remove from the microwave and stir in the almond flour until a dough forms.

Place the dough between 2 parchment paper pieces and, with a rolling pin, roll to flatten it.

Remove the upper parchment paper piece.

Divide the rolled dough into four pieces.

Place one tablespoon of pate onto each dough piece and top with one steak piece.

Cover each steak piece with dough completely.

Arrange the covered steak pieces onto the prepared baking sheet in a single layer.

Baking time: 20-30 minutes

Serve warm.

Nutrition: Calories: 412 Fat: 15.6g Fiber: 9.1g Carbohydrates:4.9 g Protein: 18.5g

16. KETO CROQUE MONSIEUR

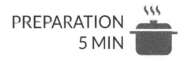

PREPARATION
5 MIN

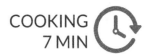

COOKING
7 MIN

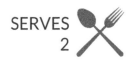

SERVES
2

INGREDIENTS

- ▸ 2 eggs
- ▸ 25 g of grated cheese
- ▸ 25 g of ham 1 large slice
- ▸ 40 ml of cream
- ▸ 40 ml of mascarpone
- ▸ 30 g of butter
- ▸ Pepper and salt
- ▸ Basil leaves, optional, to garnish

DIRECTIONS

Carefully crack eggs in a neat bowl, add some salt and pepper

Add the cream, mascarpone, grated cheese, and stir together

Melt the butter over medium heat. The butter must not turn brown

Once the butter has melted, set the heat to low

Add half of the omelette mixture to the frying pan and then immediately place the slice of ham on it

Now pour the rest of the omelette mixture over the ham and then immediately put a lid on it

Allow it to fry for 2-3 minutes over low

heat until the top is slightly firmer

Slide the omelette onto the lid to turn the omelette

Then put the omelette back in the frying pan to fry for another 1-2 minutes on the other side (still on low heat), then put the lid back on the pan

Don't let the omelette cook for too long!

It does not matter if it is still liquid

Garnish with a few basil leaves if necessary

Nutrition: Calories: 479 kcal Protein: 16 g Fats: 45 g Net carbohydrates: 4 g

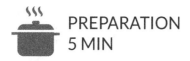

**PREPARATION
5 MIN**

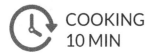

**COOKING
10 MIN**

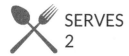

**SERVES
2**

17. KETO WRAPS WITH CREAM CHEESE AND SALMON

INGREDIENTS

- 80 g of cream cheese
- 1 tablespoon of dill or other fresh herbs
- 30 g of smoked salmon
- 1 egg
- 15 g of butter
- Pinch of cayenne pepper
- Pepper and salt

DIRECTIONS

Beat the egg well in a bowl. With 1 egg, you can make two thin wraps in a small frying pan.

Melt the butter over medium heat in a small frying pan.

Once the butter has melted, add half of the beaten egg to the pan.

Move the pan back and forth so that the entire bottom is covered with a very thin layer of egg. Turn down the heat!

Carefully loosen the egg on the edges with a silicone spatula and turn the wafer-thin omelette as soon as the egg is no longer dripping (about 45 seconds to 1 minute).

You can do this by sliding it onto a lid or plate and then sliding it back into the pan.

Let the other side be cooked for about 30 seconds and then remove from the pan.

The omelette must be nice and light yellow.

Repeat for the rest of the beaten egg

Once the omelettes are ready, let them cool on a cutting board or plate and make the filling

Cut the dill into small pieces and put in a bowl

Add the cream cheese, the salmon cut into small pieces, and mix together. Add a tiny bit of cayenne pepper and mix well. Taste immediately and then season with salt and pepper.

Spread a layer on the wrap and roll it up. Cut the wrap in half and keep in the fridge until you are ready to eat it.

Nutrition: Calories: 237 kcal Carbohydrates: 14.7 g Protein: 15 g Fat: 5 g

18. SESAME PORK WITH GREEN BEANS

PREPARATION
5 MIN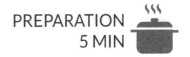

COOKING
10 MIN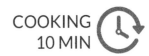

SERVES
2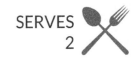

INGREDIENTS

- ▸ 2 boneless pork chops
- ▸ Pink Himalayan salt
- ▸ Freshly ground black pepper
- ▸ 2 tablespoons toasted sesame oil, divided
- ▸ 2 tablespoons soy sauce
- ▸ 1 teaspoon Sriracha sauce
- ▸ 1 cup fresh green beans

. . . .

DIRECTIONS

On a cutting board, pat the pork chops dry with a paper towel. Slice the chops into strips and season with pink Himalayan salt and pepper.

In a large skillet over medium heat, heat one tablespoon of sesame oil.

Add the pork strips and cook them for 7 minutes, stirring occasionally.

In a small bowl, mix the remaining one tablespoon of sesame oil, the soy sauce, and the Sriracha sauce. Pour into the skillet with the pork.

Add the green beans to the skillet, reduce the heat to medium-low, and simmer for 3 to 5 minutes.

Divide the pork, green beans, and sauce between two wide, shallow bowls and serve.

Nutrition: Calories: 387 Fat: 15.1g Fiber: 10g Carbohydrates:4.1 g Protein:18.1 g

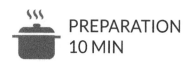 **PREPARATION**
10 MIN

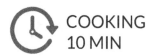 **COOKING**
10 MIN

 **SERVES**
4

19. PAN-SEARED COD WITH TOMATO HOLLANDAISE

INGREDIENTS

- ► Pan-Seared Cod
- ► 1 pound (4-fillets) wild Alaskan Cod
- ► 1 tbsp. salted butter
- ► 1 tbsp. olive oil
- ► Tomato Hollandaise
- ► 3 large egg yolks
- ► 3 tbsp. warm water
- ► 226 grams salted butter, melted
- ► 1/4 tsp. salt
- ► 1/4 tsp. black pepper

- ► 2 tbsp. tomato paste
- ► 2 tbsp. fresh lemon juice

DIRECTIONS

Season both sides of the code fillet without salt, the salt will be added in the last.

Heat a skillet over medium heat and coat with olive oil and butter.

When the butter heats up, place the cod fillet in the skillet and sear on both sides for 2-3 minutes. Baste the fish fillet with the oil and butter mixture.

You will know that the cod cooked when it easily flakes when poked with a fork.

Melt the butter in the microwave.

In a double boil, beat egg yolks with warm water until thick and creamy and start forming soft peaks. Remove the double boil from the heat, gradually adding the melted butter and stirring.

Season.

Mix in the tomato paste. Stir to combine. Pour in the water and lemon juice to lighten the sauce texture.

Nutrition: Calories: 356 Fat: 16.1g Fiber: 12.3g Carbohydrates:3.1 g Protein: 18.4g

20. CREAMY SCALLOPS

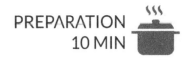

PREPARATION
10 MIN

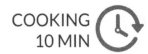

COOKING
10 MIN

SERVES
4

INGREDIENTS

- 1 lb scallops, rinse and pat dry
- 1 tsp fresh parsley, chopped
- 1/8 tsp cayenne pepper
- 2 tbsp white wine
- 1/4 cup water
- 3 tbsp heavy cream
- 1 tsp garlic, minced
- 1 tbsp butter, melted
- 1 tbsp olive oil
- Pepper
- Salt

DIRECTIONS

Season scallops with pepper and salt

Heat butter and oil in a pan over medium heat

Add scallops and sear until browned from both sides. Transfer scallops on a plate

Add garlic in the same pan and saute for 30 seconds

Add water, heavy cream, wine, cayenne pepper, and salt. Stir well and cook until sauce thickens

Return scallops to pan and stir well

Garnish with parsley and serve

Nutrition: Calories: 202 kcal Fat: 11.4 g Carbohydrates: 3.5 g Sugar: 0.1 g Protein: 19.4 g Cholesterol: 60 mg

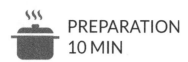
PREPARATION
10 MIN

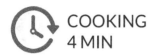
COOKING
4 MIN

SERVES
4

21. PERFECT PAN-SEARED SCALLOPS

INGREDIENTS

- ▸ 1 lb scallops, rinse and pat dry
- ▸ 1 tbsp olive oil
- ▸ 2 tbsp butter
- ▸ Pepper
- ▸ Salt

• •

DIRECTIONS

Season scallops with pepper and salt

Heat butter and oil in a pan over medium heat

Add scallops and sear for 2 minutes then turn to the other side and cook for 2 minutes more

Serve and enjoy

Nutrition: Calories: 181 kcal Fat: 10.1 g Carbohydrates: 2.7 g Sugar: 0 g Protein: 19.1 g Cholesterol: 53 mg

22. EASY BAKED SHRIMP SCAMPI

PREPARATION
10 MIN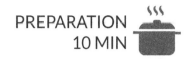

COOKING
10 MIN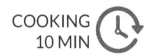

SERVES
4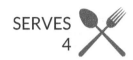

INGREDIENTS

- 2 lb shrimp, peeled
- 3/4 cup olive oil
- 2 tsp dried oregano
- 1 tbsp garlic, minced
- 1/2 cup fresh lemon juice
- 1/4 cup butter, sliced
- Pepper
- Salt

DIRECTIONS

Preheat the oven to 350 °F

Add shrimp in a baking dish

In a bowl, whisk together lemon juice, oregano, garlic, oil, pepper, salt, and pour over shrimp

Add butter on top of shrimp

Bake in preheated oven for 10 minutes or until shrimp is cooked

Serve and enjoy

Nutrition: Calories: 708 kcal Fat: 53.5 g Carbohydrates: 5.3 g Sugar: 0.7 g Protein: 52.2 g Cholesterol: 508 mg

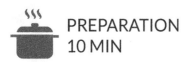

PREPARATION
10 MIN

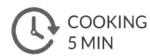

COOKING
5 MIN

SERVES
4

23. DELICIOUS BLACKENED SHRIMP

INGREDIENTS

- 1 1/2 lbs shrimp, peeled
- 1 tbsp garlic, minced
- 1 tbsp olive oil
- 1 tsp garlic powder
- 1 tsp dried oregano
- 1 tsp cumin
- 1 tbsp paprika
- 1 tbsp chili powder
- Pepper
- Salt

DIRECTIONS

In a mixing bowl, mix together garlic powder, oregano, cumin, paprika, chili powder, pepper, and salt

Add shrimp and mix until well coated. Set aside for 30 minutes

Heat oil in a pan over medium-high heat

Add shrimp and cook for 2 minutes. Turn shrimp and cook for 2 minutes more

Add garlic and cook for 30 seconds

Serve and enjoy

Nutrition: Calories 252 kcal Fat: 7.1 g Carbohydrates: 6.3 g Sugar: 0.5 g Protein: 39.6 g Cholesterol: 358 mg

PREPARATION
15 MIN
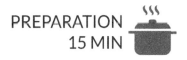

COOKING
15 MIN
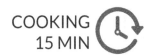

SERVES
6

24. SIGNATURE ITALIAN PORK DISH

INGREDIENTS

- 2 lb. pork tenderloins, cut into 1½-inch pieces
- ¼ C almond flour
- 1 tsp garlic salt
- Freshly ground black pepper, to taste
- 2 tbsp butter
- ½ C homemade chicken broth
- 1/3 C balsamic vinegar
- 1 tbsp capers
- 2 tsp fresh lemon zest, grated finely

DIRECTIONS

In a large bowl, add the pork pieces, flour, garlic salt, black pepper, and toss to coat well

Remove pork pieces from bowl and shake off excess flour mixture

In a large skillet, melt the butter over medium-high heat and cook the pork pieces for about 2-3 minutes per side

Add broth and vinegar and bring to a gentle boil

Reduce the heat to medium and simmer for about 3-4 minutes

With a slotted spoon, transfer the pork pieces onto a plate

In the same skillet, add the capers, lemon zest, and simmer for about 3-5 minutes or until the desired thickness of sauce

Pour sauce over pork pieces and serve

Nutrition: Calories: 373 kcal Carbohydrates: 1.8 g Protein: 46.7 g Fat: 18.6 g Sugar: 0.4 g Sodium: 231 mg Fiber: 0.7 g

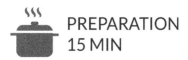

PREPARATION
15 MIN

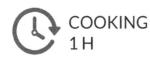

COOKING
1 H

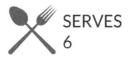

SERVES
6

25. FLAVOR PACKED PORK LOIN

INGREDIENTS

- 1/3 C. low-sodium soy sauce
- ¼ C fresh lemon juice
- 2 tsp fresh lemon zest, grated
- 1 tbs. fresh thyme, finely chopped
- 2 tbsp fresh ginger, grated
- 2 garlic cloves, chopped finely
- 2 tbsp Erythritol
- Freshly ground black pepper, to taste
- ½ tsp cayenne pepper
- 2 lb boneless pork loin

DIRECTIONS

For pork marinade: in a large baking dish, add all the ingredients except pork loin and mix until well combined

Add the pork loin and coat with the marinade generously

Refrigerate for about 24 hours

Preheat the oven to 400 °F

Remove the pork loin from marinade and arrange it into a baking dish

Cover the baking dish and bake for about 1 hour

Remove from the oven and place the pork loin onto a cutting board

With a piece of foil, cover each loin for at least 10 minutes before slicing

With a sharp knife, cut the pork loin into desired size slices and serve

Nutrition: Calories: 230 kcal Carbohydrates: 3.2 g Protein: 40.8 g Fat: 5.6 g Sugar: 1.2 g Sodium: 871 mg Fiber: 0.6 g

PREPARATION
15 MIN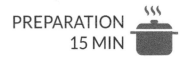

COOKING
18 MIN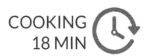

SERVES
6

26. SPICED PORK TENDERLOIN

INGREDIENTS

- ► 2 tsp fresh rosemary, minced
- ► 2 tsp fennel seeds
- ► 2 tsp coriander seeds
- ► 2 tsp caraway seeds
- ► 1 tsp cumin seeds
- ► 1 bay leaf
- ► Salt and freshly ground black pepper, to taste
- ► 2 tbsp fresh dill, chopped
- ► 1-2 lb pork tenderloins, trimmed

DIRECTIONS

For spice rub: in a spice grinder, add the seeds and bay leaf and grind until finely powdered

Add the salt and black pepper and mix

In a small bowl, reserve 2 tbsp. of spice rub

In another small bowl, mix together the remaining spice rub, and dill

Place 1 tenderloin over a piece of plastic wrap

With a sharp knife, slice through the meat to within ½-inch of the opposite side

Now, open the tenderloin like a book

Cover with another plastic wrap and with a meat pounder, gently pound into ½-inch thickness

Repeat with the remaining tenderloin

Remove the plastic wrap and spread half of the dill mixture over the center of each tenderloin

Roll each tenderloin like a cylinder

With a kitchen string, tightly tie each roll at several places

Rub each roll with the reserved spice rub generously

With 1 plastic wrap, wrap each roll and refrigerate for at least 4-6 hours.

Preheat the grill to medium-high heat. Grease the grill grate

Remove the plastic wrap from tenderloins

Place tenderloins onto the grill and cook for about 14-18 minutes, flipping occasionally

Remove from the grill and place tenderloins onto a cutting board and with a piece of foil, cover each tenderloin for at least 5-10 minutes before slicing

With a sharp knife, cut the tenderloins into desired size slices and serve

Nutrition: Calories: 313 kcal Carbohydrates: 1.4 g Protein: 45.7 g Fat: 12.6 g Sugar: 0 g Sodium: 127 mg Fiber: 0.7 g

PREPARATION
15 MIN

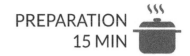

COOKING
2H 34 MIN

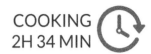

SERVES
9

27. STICKY PORK RIBS

INGREDIENTS

- ¼ C Erythritol
- 1 tbsp garlic powder
- 1 tbsp paprika
- ½ tsp red chili powder
- 4 lb pork ribs, membrane removed
- Salt and freshly ground black pepper, to taste
- 1½ tsp liquid smoke
- 1½ C sugar-free BBQ sauce

DIRECTIONS

Preheat the oven to 300 °F.

Line a large baking sheet with 2 layers of foil, shiny side out

In a bowl, add the Erythritol, garlic powder, paprika, chili powder, and mix well

Season the ribs with salt and black pepper and then, coat with the liquid smoke

Now, rub the ribs with the Erythritol mixture

Arrange the ribs onto the prepared baking sheet, meaty side down

Arrange 2 layers of foil on top of ribs and then, roll and crimp edges tightly

Bake for about 2-2½ hours or until the desired doneness

Remove the baking sheet from oven and place the ribs onto a cutting board

Now, set the oven to broiler

With a sharp knife, cut the ribs into serving sized portions and evenly coat with the barbecue sauce

Arrange the ribs onto a broiler pan, bony side up

Broil for about 1-2 minutes per side

Remove from the oven and serve hot

Nutrition: Calories: 530 kcal Carbohydrates: 2.8 g Protein: 60.4 g Fat: 40.3 g Sugar: 0.4 g Sodium: 306 mg Fiber: 0.5 g

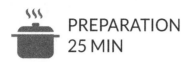

**PREPARATION
25 MIN**

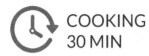

**COOKING
30 MIN**

**SERVES
2**

28. LOW-CALORIE CHEESY BROCCOLI QUICHE

INGREDIENTS

- 1/3 tablespoon butter
- Black pepper
- 4 oz broccoli
- ¼ teaspoon garlic powder
- 2 tablespoon full-fat cream
- 1/8 cup scallions
- Kosher salt
- ¼ cup cheddar cheese
- 2 eggs

DIRECTIONS

Warm-up, the oven to 360 degrees F, then grease the baking dish with butter

Put broccoli and 4 to 8 tablespoons water and place the bowl in the microwave within 3 minutes. Mix and again bake within 3 minutes

Beat the eggs in a bowl. Pour all leftover items with broccoli

Put all mixture in the baking dish. Bake within 30 minutes. Slice and serve

Nutrition: Calories: 196 kcal Fats: 14 g Carbohydrates: 5 g Proteins: 12 g Fiber: 2 g

29. LOW CARB BROCCOLI LEEK SOUP

PREPARATION
15 MIN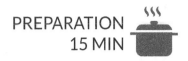

COOKING
15 MIN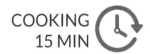

SERVES
2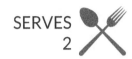

INGREDIENTS

- ½ leek
- 100 g cream cheese
- 150 g broccoli
- ½ cup heavy cream
- 1 cup of water
- ¼ tablespoon black pepper
- ½ vegetable bouillon cube
- ¼ cup basil
- 1 teaspoon garlic
- Salt

DIRECTIONS

Put water into a pan and put broccoli chopped, leek chopped, and salt.

Boil on high

Simmer on low

Put the remaining items, simmer for 1 minute. Remove

Blend the soup mixture into a blender. Serve

Nutrition: Calories: 545 kcal Fats: 50 g Carbohydrates: 10 g Proteins: 15 g

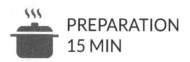

PREPARATION
15 MIN

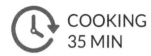

COOKING
35 MIN

SERVES
4

30. CLASSIC PORK TENDERLOIN

INGREDIENTS

- 8 bacon slices
- 2 lb. pork tenderloin
- 1 tsp. dried oregano, crushed
- 1 tsp. dried basil, crushed
- 1 tbsp. garlic powder
- 1 tsp. seasoned salt
- 3 tbsp. butter

DIRECTIONS

Preheat the oven to 400 degrees F.

Heat a large ovenproof skillet over medium-high heat and cook the bacon for about 6-7 minutes.

Transfer the bacon onto a paper towel lined plate to drain.

Then, wrap the pork tenderloin with bacon slices and secure with toothpicks.

With a sharp knife, slice the tenderloin between each bacon slice to make a medallion.

In a bowl, mix together the dried herbs, garlic powder and seasoned salt.

Now, coat the medallion with herb mixture.

With a paper towel, wipe out the skillet.

In the same skillet, melt the butter over medium-high heat and cook the pork medallion for about 4 minutes per side.

Now, transfer the skillet into the oven.

Roast for about 17-20 minutes.

Remove the wok from oven and let it cool slightly before cutting.

Cut the tenderloin into desired size slices and serve.

Nutrition: Calories: 471 Cal Fat: 19 g Carbs: 8 g Protein: 9 g Fiber: 3 g

31. SPICY KETO CHICKEN WINGS

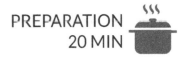

PREPARATION
20 MIN

COOKING
30 MIN

SERVES
4

INGREDIENTS

- 2 lb Chicken Wings
- 1 t Cajun Spice
- 2 t Smoked Paprika
- 0.5 t Turmeric
- Salt - Dash
- 2 t Baking Powder
- Pepper - Dash

DIRECTIONS

When you first begin the Ketogenic Diet, you may find that you won't be eating the traditional foods that may have made up a majority of your diet in the past .While this is a good thing for your health, you may feel you are missing out! The good news is that there are delicious alternatives that aren't lacking in flavor!

To start this recipe, you'll want to prep the stove to 400 °F

As this heat up, you will want to take some time to dry your chicken wings with a paper towel. This will help remove any excess moisture and get you some nice, crispy wings!

When you are all set, take out a mixing bowl and place all of the seasonings along with the baking powder

If you feel like it, you can adjust the seasoning levels however you would like

Once these are set, go ahead and throw the chicken wings in and coat evenly

If you have one, you'll want to place the wings on a wire rack that is placed over your baking tray. If not, you can just lay them across the baking sheet

Now that your chicken wings are set, you are going to pop them into the stove for thirty minutes

By the end of this time, the tops of the wings should be crispy

If they are, take them out from the oven and flip them so that you can bake the other side.

You will want to cook these for an additional thirty minutes

Finally, take the tray from the oven and allow it to cool slightly before serving up your spiced keto wings

For additional flavor, serve with any of your favorite, keto-friendly dipping sauce

Nutrition: Fats: 7 g Carbs: 1 g Proteins: 60 g Calories 299 kcal

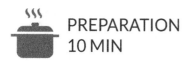

PREPARATION
10 MIN

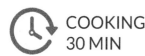

COOKING
30 MIN

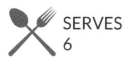

SERVES
6

32. CHEESY HAM QUICHE

INGREDIENTS

- 8 eggs
- 1 c Zucchini
- 0.5 c Shredded heavy Cream
- 1 c Ham, Diced
- 1 t Mustard
- Salt – Dash

DIRECTIONS

For this recipe, you can start off by prepping your stove to 375 and getting out a pie plate for your quiche

Next, it is time to prep the zucchini. First, you will want to go ahead and shred it into small pieces

Once this is complete, take a paper towel and gently squeeze out the excess moisture. This will help avoid a soggy quiche

When the step from above is complete, you will want to place the zucchini into your pie plate along with the cooked ham pieces and your cheese

Once these items are in place, you will want to whisk the seasonings, cream, and eggs together before pouring it over the top

Now that your quiche is set, you are going to pop the dish into your stove for about forty minutes

By the end of this time, the egg should be cooked through, and you will be able to insert a knife into the center and have it come out clean

If the quiche is cooked to your liking, take the dish from the oven and allow it to chill slightly before slicing and serving

Nutrition: Fats: 25 g Carbs: 2 g Proteins: 20 g Calories 211 kcal

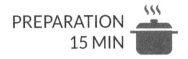

PREPARATION
15 MIN

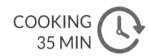

COOKING
35 MIN

SERVES
6

33. BROCCOLI AND CHICKEN CASSEROLE

INGREDIENTS

- 2 tablespoons butter
- 1/4 cup cooked bacon, crumbled
- 21/2 cups cheddar cheese, shredded and divided
- 4 ounces cream cheese, softened
- 1/4 cup heavy whipping cream
- 1/2 pack ranch seasoning mix
- 2/3 cup homemade chicken broth
- 11/2 cups small broccoli florets
- 2 cups cooked grass-fed chicken breast, shredded

DIRECTIONS

Preheat your oven to 350°F.

Arrange a rack in the upper portion of the oven.

For the chicken mixture: In a large wok, melt the butter over low heat.

Add the bacon, 1/2 cup of cheddar cheese, cream cheese, heavy whipping cream, ranch seasoning, and broth, and with a wire whisk, beat until well combined.

Cook for about 5 minutes, stirring frequently.

Meanwhile, in a microwave-safe dish, place the broccoli and microwave until desired tenderness is achieved.

In the wok, add the chicken and broccoli and mix until well combined.

Remove from the heat and transfer the mixture into a casserole dish.

Top the chicken mixture with the remaining cheddar cheese.

Bake for about 25 minutes.

Now, set the oven to broiler.

Broil the chicken mixture for about 2–3 minutes or until cheese is bubbly.

Serve hot.

Nutrition: Calories: 431 Fat: 10.5g Fiber: 9.1g Carbohydrates:4.9 g Protein: 14.1g

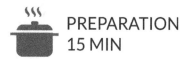

PREPARATION
15 MIN

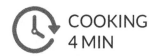

COOKING
4 MIN

SERVES
4

34. LAMB CHOPS AND HERB BUTTER

INGREDIENTS

- 8 lamb chops;
- 1 tbsp each:
- Olive oil
- Butter
- Pepper
- Salt;
- **For the herb butter:**
- 5 ounces butter
- 1 clove garlic
- Half tbsp. garlic powder

- 4 tbsps parsley
- 1 tsp lemon juice
- 1-third tsp salt

DIRECTIONS

Season the lamb chops with pepper and salt

Warm-up olive oil and butter in an iron skillet. Add the lamb chops. Fry within four minutes

Mix all the listed items for the herb butter in a bowl. Cool

Serve with herb butter

Nutrition: Calories: 722.3 kcal Protein: 42.3 g Carbs: 0.4 g Fat: 61.5 g Fiber: 0.4 g

35. PORK CHOPS IN BLUE CHEESE SAUCE

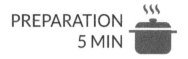

PREPARATION
5 MIN

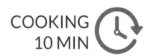

COOKING
10 MIN

SERVES
2

INGREDIENTS

- ▶ 2 boneless pork chops
- ▶ Pink Himalayan salt
- ▶ Freshly ground black pepper
- ▶ 2 tablespoons butter
- ▶ 1/3 cup blue cheese crumbles
- ▶ 1/3 cup heavy (whipping) cream
- ▶ 1/3 cup sour cream

DIRECTIONS

Dry the pork chops and season with pink Himalayan salt and pepper.

In a medium skillet over medium heat, melt the butter. When the butter melts and is very hot, add the pork chops and sear on each side for 3 minutes.

The pork chops must be transferred to a plate and let rest for 3 to 5 minutes.

In a preheated pan, melt the blue cheese crumbles, frequently stirring so they don't burn.

Add the cream and the sour cream to the pan with the blue cheese. Let simmer for a few minutes, stirring occasionally.

For an extra kick of flavor in the sauce, pour the pork-chop pan juice into the cheese mixture and stir. Let simmer while the pork chops are resting.

Put the pork chops on two plates, pour the blue cheese sauce over the top of each, and serve.

Nutrition: Calories: 434 Fat: 14.1g Fiber: 11.3g Carbohydrates:3.1 g Protein: 17.5g

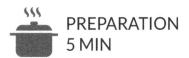 **PREPARATION**
5 MIN

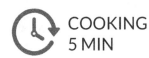 **COOKING**
5 MIN

 **SERVES**
4

36. BUTTERED COD

INGREDIENTS

- ► 1 ½ lb cod fillets, sliced
- ► 6 tablespoons butter, sliced
- ► ¼ teaspoon garlic powder
- ► ¾ teaspoon ground paprika
- ► Salt and pepper to taste
- ► Lemon slices
- ► Chopped parsley

DIRECTIONS

Mix the garlic powder, paprika, salt, and pepper in a bowl

Season cod pieces with seasoning mixture

Add 2 tablespoons butter in a pan over medium heat

Let half of the butter melt

Add the cod and cook for 2 minutes per side

Top with the remaining slices of butter

Cook for 3 to 4 minutes

Garnish with parsley and lemon slices before serving

Nutrition: Calories: 295 kcal Total Fat: 19 g Saturated Fat: 11 g Cholesterol: 128 mg Sodium: 236 mg Total Carbohydrate: 1.5 g Dietary Fiber: 0.7 g Total Sugars: 0.3 g Protein: 30.7 g Potassium: 102 mg

PREPARATION
10 MIN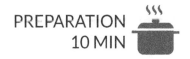

COOKING
22 MIN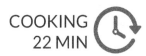

SERVES
4

37. SALMON WITH RED CURRY SAUCE

INGREDIENTS

- ▸ 4 salmon fillets
- ▸ 2 tablespoons olive oil
- ▸ Salt and pepper to taste
- ▸ 1 ½ tablespoon red curry paste
- ▸ 1 tablespoon fresh ginger, chopped
- ▸ 14 oz coconut cream
- ▸ 1 ½ tablespoons fish sauce

• •

DIRECTIONS

Preheat your oven to 350 °F.

Cover baking sheet with foil

Brush both sides of salmon fillets with olive oil and season with salt and pepper

Place the salmon fillets on the baking sheet

Bake salmon in the oven for 20 minutes

In a pan over medium heat, mix the curry paste, ginger, coconut cream, and fish sauce

Sprinkle with salt and pepper

Simmer for 2 minutes

Pour the sauce over the salmon before serving

Nutrition: Calories: 553 kcal Total Fat: 43.4 g Saturated Fat: 24.1 g Cholesterol: 78 mg Sodium: 908 mg Total Carbohydrate: 7.9 g Dietary Fiber: 2.4 g Total Sugars: 3.6 g Protein: 37.3 g Potassium: 982 mg

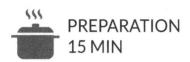

PREPARATION
15 MIN

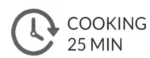

COOKING
25 MIN

SERVES
6

38. SALMON TERIYAKI

INGREDIENTS

- 3 tablespoons sesame oil
- 2 teaspoons fish sauce
- 3 tablespoons coconut amino
- 2 teaspoons ginger, grated
- 4 cloves garlic, crushed
- 2 tablespoons xylitol
- 1 tablespoon green lime juice
- 2 teaspoons green lime zest
- Cayenne pepper to taste
- 6 salmon fillets

- 1 teaspoon arrowroot starch
- ¼ cup of water
- Sesame seeds

DIRECTIONS

Preheat your oven to 400 °F

Combine the sesame oil, fish sauce, coconut amino, ginger, garlic, xylitol, green lime juice, zest, and cayenne pepper in a mixing bowl

Create 6 packets using foil

Add half of the marinade in the packets

Add the salmon inside

Place in the baking sheet and cook for about 20 to 25 minutes

Add the remaining sauce in a pan over medium heat

Dissolve the arrowroot in water and add to the sauce

Simmer until the sauce has thickened

Place the salmon on a serving platter and pour the sauce on top

Sprinkle sesame seeds on top before serving

Nutrition: Calories: 312 kcal Total Fat: 17.9 g Saturated Fat: 2.6 g Cholesterol: 78 mg Sodium: 242 mg Total Carbohydrate: 3.5 g Dietary Fiber: 0.1 g Total Sugars: 0.1 g Protein: 34.8 g Potassium: 706 mg

39. GROUND BEEF STROGANOFF

PREPARATION
10 MIN
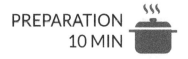

COOKING
15 MIN
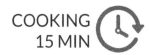

SERVES
4
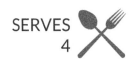

INGREDIENTS

- ▶ 2 tbsp. butter
- ▶ 1 clove minced garlic
- ▶ 1 pound 80% lean ground beef
- ▶ Salt and pepper, to taste
- ▶ 10 oz(228g) sliced mushrooms
- ▶ 2 tbsp. water
- ▶ 1 cup sour cream
- ▶ 1 tbsp. fresh lemon juice
- ▶ 1 tbsp. fresh chopped parsley

DIRECTIONS

The butter must be added to a pan. When the butter has melted and stops foaming, add the minced garlic to the skillet.

Cook the garlic until fragrant, then mix in the ground beef—season with salt and pepper.

Cook the ground beef until no longer pink; break up the grounds with a wooden spoon.

Add the water and mushrooms to the pan and cook over medium heat.

Cook until the liquid has reduced halfway, and the mushrooms are tender. Set the cooked mushrooms aside.

Reduce the heat, then whisk the sour cream and paprika into the skillet.

Stir in the cooked beef and mushrooms into the pan and combine. Stir in the lemon juice and parsley.

Nutrition: Calories: 380 Fat: 15.1g Fiber: 3.6g Carbohydrates:12.3 g Protein: 15.4g

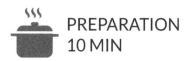

PREPARATION
10 MIN

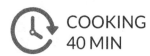

COOKING
40 MIN

SERVES
8

40. CHICKEN CASSEROLE

INGREDIENTS

- 1 lb. boneless chicken breasts, cut into 1" cubes
- 2 tablespoons. butter
- 4 tablespoons. green pesto
- 1 cup heavy whipping cream
- ¼ cup green bell peppers, diced
- 1 cup feta cheese, diced
- 1 garlic clove, minced
- Salt and pepper to taste

DIRECTIONS

Preheat your oven to 400 °F

Season the chicken with salt and pepper then batch fry in the butter until golden brown

Place the fried chicken pieces in a baking dish. Add the feta cheese, garlic, and bell peppers

Combine the pesto and heavy cream in a bowl. Pour on top of the chicken mixture and spread with a spatula

Bake for 30 minutes or until the casserole is light brown around the edges

Servings warm

Can be refrigerated for up to 5 days and frozen for 2 weeks

Nutrition: Calories: 294 kcal Carbs: 1.7 g Fat: 22.7 g Protein: 20.1 g

CHAPTER 8: DINNER RECIPES

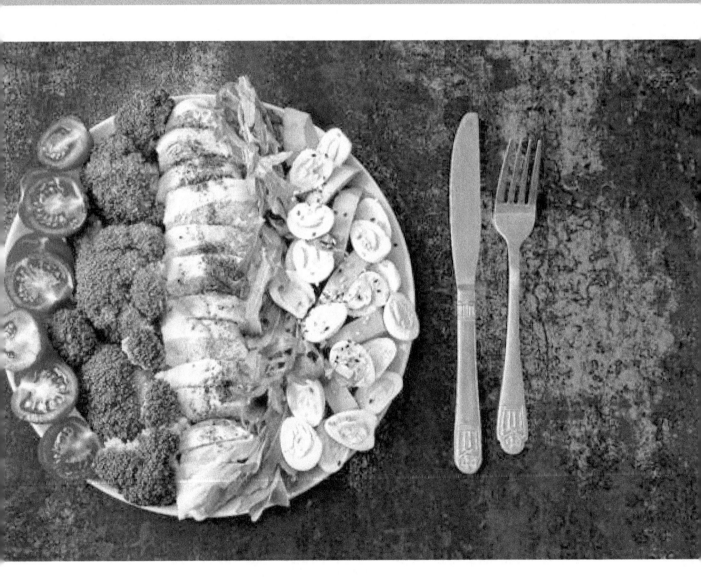

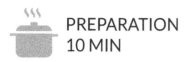

PREPARATION
10 MIN

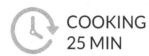

COOKING
25 MIN

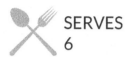

SERVES
6

41. KORMA CURRY

INGREDIENTS

- 3-pound chicken breast, skinless, boneless
- 1 teaspoon garam masala
- 1 teaspoon curry powder
- 1 tablespoon apple cider vinegar
- ½ coconut cream
- 1 cup organic almond milk
- 1 teaspoon ground coriander
- ¾ teaspoon ground cardamom
- ½ teaspoon ginger powder
- ¼ teaspoon cayenne pepper
- ¾ teaspoon ground cinnamon
- 1 tomato, diced
- 1 teaspoon avocado oil
- ½ cup of water

DIRECTIONS

Chop the chicken breast and put it in the saucepan.

Add avocado oil and start to cook it over medium heat.

Sprinkle the chicken with garam masala, curry powder, apple cider vinegar, ground coriander, cardamom, ginger powder, cayenne pepper, ground cinnamon, and diced tomato. Mix up the ingredients carefully.

Cook them for 10 minutes.

Add water, coconut cream, and almond milk. Saute the meat for 10 minutes more.

Nutrition: Calories: 440 kcal Fat: 32 g Fiber: 4 g Carbohydrates: 28 g Protein: 8 g

42. CREAMY ZOODLES

PREPARATION
15 MIN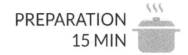

COOKING
10 MIN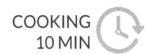

SERVES
4

INGREDIENTS

- ▸ 11/4 cups heavy whipping cream
- ▸ 1/4 cup mayonnaise
- ▸ Salt and ground black pepper, as required
- ▸ 30 ounces zucchini, spiralized with blade C
- ▸ 3 ounces Parmesan cheese, grated
- ▸ 2 tablespoons fresh mint leaves
- ▸ 2 tablespoons butter, melted

DIRECTIONS

The heavy cream must be added to a pan then bring to a boil.

Lower the heat to low and cook until reduced in half.

Put in the pepper, mayo, and salt; cook until mixture is warm enough.

Add the zucchini noodles and gently stir to combine.

Stir in the Parmesan cheese.

Divide the zucchini noodles onto four serving plates and Immediately drizzle with the melted butter.

Serve immediately.

Nutrition: Calories: 241 Fat: 11.4g Fiber: 7.5g Carbohydrates:3.1 g Protein: 5.1g

PREPARATION
30 MIN

COOKING
50 MIN

SERVES
4

43. CHEESY BACON SQUASH SPAGHETTI

INGREDIENTS

- 2 pounds spaghetti squash
- 2 pounds bacon
- 1/2 cup of butter
- 2 cups of shredded parmesan cheese
- Salt
- Black pepper

DIRECTIONS

Let the oven preheat to 375F.

Trim or remove each stem of spaghetti squash, slice into rings no more than an inch wide, and take out the seeds.

Lay the sliced rings down on the baking sheet, bake for 40-45 minutes.

It is ready when the strands separate easily when a fork is used to scrape it. Let it cool.

Cook sliced up bacon until crispy. Take out and let it cool.

Take off the shell on each ring, separate each strand with a fork, and put them in a bowl.

Heat the strands in a microwave to get them warm, then put in butter and stir around till the butter melts.

Pour in parmesan cheese and bacon crumbles, and add salt and pepper to your taste.

Enjoy.

Nutrition: Calories: 398 Fat: 12.5g Fiber: 9.4g Carbohydrates:4.1 g Protein: 5.1g

44. STUFFED PORTOBELLO MUSHROOMS

PREPARATION
10 MIN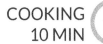

COOKING
10 MIN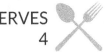

SERVES
4

INGREDIENTS

- 2 portobello mushrooms
- 1 cup spinach, chopped, steamed
- 2 oz artichoke hearts, drained, chopped
- 1 tablespoon coconut cream
- 1 tablespoon cream cheese
- 1 teaspoon minced garlic
- 1 tablespoon fresh cilantro, chopped
- 3 oz Cheddar cheese, grated
- ½ teaspoon ground black pepper
- 2 tablespoons olive oil
- ½ teaspoon salt

DIRECTIONS

Sprinkle mushrooms with olive oil and place in the tray

Transfer the tray to the preheated to 360 °F oven and broil them for 5 minutes

Meanwhile, blend artichoke hearts, coconut cream, cream cheese, minced garlic, and chopped cilantro

Add grated cheese to the mixture and sprinkle with ground black pepper and salt

Fill the broiled mushrooms with the cheese mixture and cook them for 5 minutes more. Serve the mushrooms only hot

Nutrition: Calories: 135.2 kcal Total Fat: 5.5 g Cholesterol: 16.4 mg Sodium:698.1mg- Potassium: 275.3 mg Total Carbohydrate: 8.4 g Protein: 14.8 g

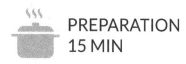

PREPARATION
15 MIN

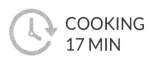

COOKING
17 MIN

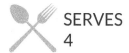

SERVES
4

45. PESTO FLAVORED STEAK

INGREDIENTS

- ¼ C. fresh oregano, chopped
- 1½ tbsp garlic, minced
- 1 tbsp fresh lemon peel, grated
- ½ tsp red pepper flakes, crushed
- Salt and freshly ground black pepper, to taste
- 1 lb (1-inch thick) grass-fed boneless beef top sirloin steak
- 1 C pesto
- ¼ C feta cheese, crumbled

DIRECTIONS

Preheat the gas grill to medium heat. Lightly, grease the grill grate

In a bowl, add the oregano, garlic, lemon peel, red pepper flakes, salt, black pepper, and mix well.

Rub the garlic mixture onto the steak evenly

Place the steak onto the grill and cook, covered for about 12-17 minutes, flipping occasionally

Remove from the grill and place the steak onto a cutting board for about 5 minutes

With a sharp knife, cut the steak into desired sized slices

Divide the steak slices and pesto onto serving plates and serve with the topping of the feta cheese

Nutrition: Calories: 226 kcal Carbohydrates: 6.8 g Protein: 40.5 g Fat: 7.6 g Sugar: 0.7 g Sodium: 579 mg Fiber: 2.2 g

46. FLAWLESS GRILLED STEAK

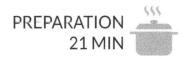

PREPARATION
21 MIN

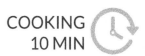

COOKING
10 MIN

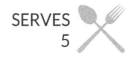

SERVES
5

INGREDIENTS

- ½ tsp dried thyme, crushed
- ½ tsp dried oregano, crushed
- 1 tsp red chili powder
- ½ tsp ground cumin
- ¼ tsp garlic powder
- Salt and freshly ground black pepper, to taste
- 1½ lb grass-fed flank steak, trimmed
- ¼ C Monterrey Jack cheese, crumbled

DIRECTIONS

In a large bowl, add the dried herbs and spices and mix well

Add the steaks and rub with mixture generously

Set aside for about 15-20 minutes

Preheat the grill to medium heat. Grease the grill grate

Place the steak onto the grill over medium coals and cook for about 17-21 minutes, flipping once halfway through

Remove the steak from the grill and place onto a cutting board for about 10 minutes before slicing

With a sharp knife, cut the steak into desired sized slices

Top with the cheese and serve

Nutrition: Calories: 271 kcal Carbohydrates: 0.7 g Protein: 38.3 g Fat: 11.8 g Sugar: 0.1 g Sodium: 119 mg Fiber: 0.3 g

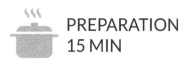

PREPARATION
15 MIN

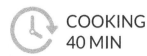

COOKING
40 MIN

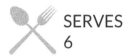

SERVES
6

47. BRUSSELS SPROUTS WITH BACON

INGREDIENTS

▶ 16 oz bacon
▶ 16 oz brussel sprouts
▶ Black pepper

DIRECTIONS

Warm the oven to reach 400 °F

Slice the bacon into small lengthwise pieces. Put the sprouts and bacon with pepper

Bake within 35 to 40 minutes. Serve

Nutrition: Carbohydrates: 3.9 g Protein: 7.9 g Total Fats: 6.9 g Calories: 113 kcal

48. KALUA PORK WITH CABBAGE

PREPARATION
10 MIN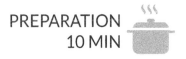

COOKING
8 H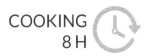

SERVES
4

INGREDIENTS

- ▸ 1-pound boneless pork butt roast
- ▸ Pink Himalayan salt
- ▸ Freshly ground black pepper
- ▸ 1 tablespoon smoked paprika or Liquid Smoke
- ▸ 1/2 cup of water
- ▸ 1/2 head cabbage, chopped

· ·

DIRECTIONS

With the crock insert in place, preheat the slow cooker to low.

Generously season the pork roast with pink Himalayan salt, pepper, and smoked paprika.

Place the pork roast in the slow-cooker insert, and add the water.

Cover and cook on low for 7 hours.

Transfer the cooked pork roast to a plate. Put the chopped cabbage in the bottom of the slow cooker, and put the pork roast back in on the cabbage.

Cover and cook the cabbage and pork roast for 1 hour.

Remove the pork roast from the slow cooker and place it on a baking sheet. Use two forks to shred the pork.

Serve the shredded pork hot with the cooked cabbage.

Reserve the liquid from the slow cooker to remoisten the pork and cabbage when reheating leftovers.

Nutrition: Calories: 451kcal Fat: 19.3g Fiber: 11.2g Carbohydrates:2.1 g Protein: 14.3g

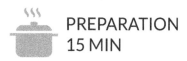

PREPARATION
15 MIN

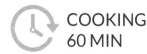

COOKING
60 MIN

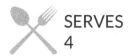

SERVES
4

49. COFFEE BBQ PORK BELLY

INGREDIENTS

- 1.5 cup beef stock
- 2 lb pork belly
- 4 tbsp olive oil
- Low-carb barbecue dry rub
- 2 tbsp instant Espresso Powder

DIRECTIONS

Set the oven at 350 °F

Heat-up the beef stock in a small saucepan

Mix in the dry barbecue rub and espresso powder

Put the pork belly, skin side up in a shallow dish and drizzle half of the oil over the top

Put the hot stock around the pork belly. Bake within 45 minutes

Sear each slice within three minutes per side. Serve

Nutrition: Net Carbohydrates: 2.6 g Protein: 24 g Total Fats: 68 g Calories: 644 kcal

50. GARLIC & THYME LAMB CHOPS

PREPARATION
15 MIN
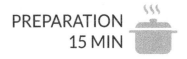

COOKING
10 MIN
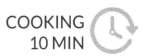

SERVES
6
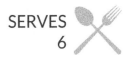

INGREDIENTS

- 6 - 4 oz lamb chops
- 4 whole garlic cloves
- 2 thyme sprigs
- 1 tsp ground thyme
- 3 tbsp olive oil

DIRECTIONS

Warm-up a skillet. Put the olive oil. Rub the chops with the spices

Put the chops in the skillet with the garlic and sprigs of thyme

Sauté within 3 to 4 minutes and serve

Nutrition: Net Carbohydrates: 1 g Protein: 14 g Total Fats: 21 g Calories: 252 kcal

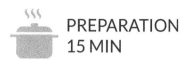

PREPARATION
15 MIN

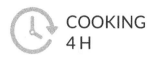

COOKING
4 H

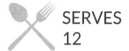

SERVES
12

51. JAMAICAN JERK PORK ROAST

INGREDIENTS

- ▶ 1 tbsp olive oil
- ▶ 4 lb pork shoulder
- ▶ 0.5 cup beef Broth
- ▶ 0.25 cup Jamaican Jerk spice blend

DIRECTIONS

Rub the roast well the oil and the jerk spice blend. Sear the roast on all sides. Put the beef broth

Simmer within four hours on low. Shred and serve

Nutrition: Net Carbohydrates: 0 g Protein: 23 g Total Fats: 20 g Calories: 282 kcal

52. KETO MEATBALLS

PREPARATION
15 MIN
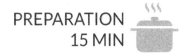

COOKING
20 MIN
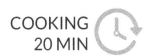

SERVES
10
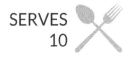

INGREDIENTS

- 1 egg
- 0.5 cup grated parmesan
- 0.5 cup shredded mozzarella
- 1 lb ground beef
- 1 tbsp garlic

DIRECTIONS

Warm-up the oven to reach 400 °F.
Combine all of the fixings

Shape into meatballs. Bake within 18-20
minutes. Cool and serve

Nutrition: Net Carbohydrates: 0.7 g Protein: 12.2 g Total Fats: 10.9 g Calories: 153 kcal

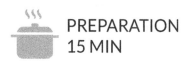

PREPARATION
15 MIN

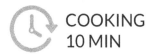

COOKING
10 MIN

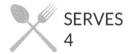

SERVES
4

53. MIXED VEGETABLE PATTIES - INSTANT POT

INGREDIENTS

▸ 1 cup cauliflower florets
▸ 1 bag vegetables
▸ 1.5 cup Water
▸ 1 cup flax meal
▸ 2 tbsp olive oil

DIRECTIONS

Steam the veggies to the steamer basket within 4 to 5 minutes.

Mash in the flax meal.

Shape into 4 patties

Cook the patties within 3 minutes per side.

Serve

Nutrition: Net Carbohydrates: 3 g Protein: 4 g Total Fats: 10 g Calories: 220 kcal

54. ROASTED LEG OF LAMB

PREPARATION
15 MIN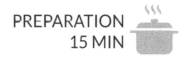

COOKING
1H 30 MIN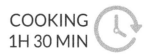

SERVES
6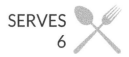

INGREDIENTS

- 0.5 cup reduced-sodium beef broth
- 2 lb lamb leg
- 6 garlic cloves
- 1 tbsp rosemary leaves
- 1 tsp black pepper

DIRECTIONS

Warm-up oven temperature to 400 °F

Put the lamb in the pan and put the broth and seasonings

Roast 30 minutes and lower the heat to 350 °F. Cook within one hour

Cool and serve

Nutrition: Net Carbohydrates: 1 g Protein: 22 g Total Fats: 14 g Calories: 223 kcal

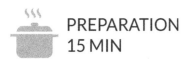

PREPARATION
15 MIN

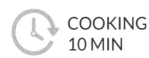

COOKING
10 MIN

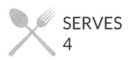

SERVES
4

55. MONGOLIAN BEEF

INGREDIENTS

- 1 lb. grass-fed flank steak, cut into thin slices against the grain
- 2 tsp. arrowroot starch
- Salt, to taste
- ¼ C avocado oil
- 1 (1-inch) piece fresh ginger, grated
- 4 garlic cloves, minced
- ½ tsp red pepper flakes, crushed
- ¼ C water
- 1/3 C low-sodium soy sauce
- 1 tsp red boat fish sauce
- 3 scallions, sliced
- 1 tsp sesame seeds

DIRECTIONS

In a bowl, add the steak slices, arrowroot starch, salt, and toss to coat well

In a larger skillet, heat oil over medium-high heat and cook the steak slices for about 1½ minutes per side

With a slotted spoon, transfer the steak slices onto a plate

Drain the oil from the skillet but leaving about 1 tbsp. inside

In the same skillet, add the ginger, garlic, red pepper flakes, and sauté for about 1 minute

Add the water, soy sauce, fish sauce, and stir to combine well

Stir in the cooked steak slices and simmer for about 3 minutes

Stir in the scallions and simmer for about 2 minutes

Remove from the heat and serve hot with the garnishing of sesame seeds

Nutrition: Calories: 266 kcal Carbohydrates: 5.7 g Protein: 34 g Fat: 11.7 g Sugar: 1.7 g Sodium: 1350 mg Fiber: 1.2 g

56. LETTUCE SALAD

PREPARATION
10 MIN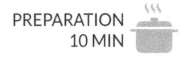

COOKING
0 MIN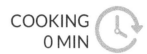

SERVES
1

INGREDIENTS

▸ 1 cup Romaine lettuce, roughly chopped
▸ 3 oz seitan, chopped
▸ 1 tablespoon avocado oil
▸ 1 teaspoon sunflower seeds
▸ 1 teaspoon lemon juice
▸ 1 egg, boiled, peeled
▸ 2 oz Cheddar cheese, shredded

DIRECTIONS

Place lettuce in the salad bowl. Add chopped seitan and shredded cheese

Then chop the egg roughly and add in the salad bowl too

Mix up together lemon juice with the avocado oil

Sprinkle the salad with the oil mixture and sunflower seeds. Don't stir the salad before serving

Nutrition: Calories: 20 kcal Total Fat: 0.2 g Cholesterol: 0 mg Sodium: 31 mg Potassium: 241 mg Total Carbohydrates: 4.2 g Protein: 1.2 g

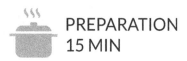

PREPARATION
15 MIN

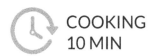

COOKING
10 MIN

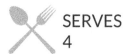

SERVES
4

57. GRAIN-FREE CREAMY NOODLES

INGREDIENTS

▶ 1¼ C heavy whipping cream
▶ ¼ C mayonnaise
▶ Salt and freshly ground black pepper, to taste
▶ 30 oz zucchini, spiralized with blade C
▶ 4 organic egg yolks
▶ 3 oz Parmesan cheese, grated
▶ 2 tbsp fresh parsley, chopped
▶ 2 tbsp butter, melted

DIRECTIONS

In a pan, add the heavy cream and bring to a boil

Reduce the heat to low and cook until reduced

Add the mayonnaise, salt, black pepper, and cook until the mixture is warm enough

Add the zucchini noodles and gently, stir to combine

Immediately, remove from the heat

Place the zucchini noodles mixture onto 4 serving plates evenly and immediately, top with the egg yolks, followed by the parmesan and parsley

Drizzle with hot melted butter and serve

Nutrition: Calories: 427 kcal Carbohydrates: 9 g Protein: 13 g Fat: 39.1 g Sugar: 3.8 g Sodium: 412 mg Fiber: 2.4 g

58. MEAT-FREE ZOODLES STROGANOFF

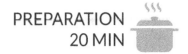

PREPARATION
20 MIN

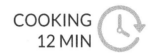

COOKING
12 MIN

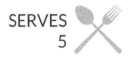

SERVES
5

INGREDIENTS

- **For Mushroom Sauce:**
- 1½ tbsp. butter
- 1 large garlic clove, minced
- 1¼ C fresh button mushrooms, sliced
- ¼ C homemade vegetable broth
- ¼ C cream
- Salt and freshly ground black pepper, to taste;
- **For Zucchini Noodles:**
- 3 large zucchinis, spiralized with blade C

- ¼ C fresh parsley leaves, chopped

DIRECTIONS

In a large bowl, add the pork pieces, flour, garlic salt, black pepper, and toss to coat well

Remove pork pieces from bowl and shake off excess flour mixture

In a large skillet, melt the butter over medium-high heat and cook the pork pieces for about 2-3 minutes per side

Add broth and vinegar and bring to a gentle boil

Reduce the heat to medium and simmer for about 3-4 minutes

With a slotted spoon, transfer the pork pieces onto a plate

In the same skillet, add the capers, lemon zest, and simmer for about 3-5 minutes or until the desired thickness of sauce

Pour sauce over pork pieces and serve

Nutrition: Calories: 77 kcal Carbohydrates: 7.9 g Protein: 3.4 g Fat: 4.6 g Sugar: 4 g Sodium: 120 mg Fiber: 2.4 g

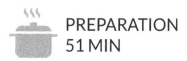

PREPARATION
51 MIN

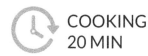

COOKING
20 MIN

SERVES
4

59. EYE-CATCHING VEGGIES

INGREDIENTS

- ¼ C butter
- 6 scallions, sliced
- 1 lb fresh white mushrooms, sliced
- 1 C tomatoes, crushed
- Salt and freshly ground black pepper, to taste
- 2 tbsp feta cheese, crumbled

DIRECTIONS

In a large pan, melt the butter over medium-low heat and sauté the scallion for about 2 minutes

Add the mushrooms and sauté for about 5-7 minutes

Stir in the tomatoes and cook for about 8-10 minutes, stirring occasionally

Stir in the salt and black pepper and remove from the heat

Serve with the topping of feta

Nutrition: Calories: 160 kcal Carbohydrates: 7.4 g Protein: 5.5 g Fat: 13.5 g Sugar: 3.9 g Sodium: 211 mg Fiber: 2.3 g

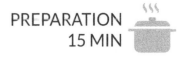

PREPARATION
15 MIN

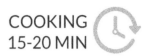

COOKING
15-20 MIN

60. CHICKEN SCHNITZEL

SERVES
4

INGREDIENTS

- 1 tbsp. chopped fresh parsley
- 4 garlic cloves, minced
- 1 tbsp. plain vinegar
- 1 tbsp. coconut aminos
- 2 tsp. sugar-free maple syrup
- 2 tsp. chili pepper
- Salt and black pepper to taste
- 6 tbsp. coconut oil
- 1 lb. asparagus, hard stems removed
- 4 chicken breasts, skin-on and boneless

- 2 cups grated Mexican cheese blend
- 1 tbsp. mixed sesame seeds
- 1 cup almond flour
- 4 eggs, beaten
- 6 tbsp. avocado oil
- 1 tsp. chili flakes for garnish

DIRECTIONS

In a bowl, whisk the parsley, garlic, vinegar, coconut aminos, maple syrup, chili pepper, salt, and black pepper. Set aside.

Heat the coconut oil in a large skillet and stir-fry the asparagus for 8 to 10 minutes or until tender. Remove the asparagus into a large bowl and toss with the vinegar mixture. Set aside for serving.

Cover the chicken breasts in plastic wraps and use a meat tenderizer to pound the chicken until flattened to 2-inch thickness gently.

On a plate, mix the Mexican cheese blend and sesame seeds. Dredge the chicken pieces in the almond flour, dip in the egg on both sides, and generously coat in the seed mix.

Heat the avocado oil. Cook the chicken until golden brown and cooked within.

Divide the asparagus onto four serving plates, place a chicken on each, and garnish with the chili flakes. Serve warm.

Nutrition: Calories: 451 Fat: 18.5g Fiber: 12.9g Carbohydrates:5.9 g Protein: 19.5g

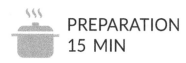

PREPARATION
15 MIN

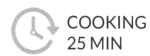

COOKING
25 MIN

SERVES
5

61. CHICKEN PARMIGIANA

INGREDIENTS

- 5 (6-ounce) grass-fed skinless, boneless chicken breasts
- 1 large organic egg, beaten
- 1/2 cup superfine blanched almond flour
- 1/4 cup Parmesan cheese, grated
- 1/2 teaspoon dried parsley
- 1/2 teaspoon paprika
- 1/2 teaspoon garlic powder
- Salt and ground black pepper, as required
- 1/4 cup olive oil
- 1 cup sugar-free tomato sauce
- 5 ounces mozzarella cheese, thinly sliced
- 2 tablespoons fresh parsley, chopped

DIRECTIONS

Preheat your oven to 375°F.

Arrange one chicken breast between 2 pieces of parchment paper.

With a meat mallet, pound the chicken breast into a 1/2-inch thickness

Repeat with the remaining chicken breasts.

Add the beaten egg into a shallow dish.

Place the almond flour, Parmesan, parsley, spices, salt, and black pepper in another shallow dish, and mix well.

Dip chicken breasts into the whipped egg and then coat with the flour mixture.

Heat the oil in a deep wok over medium-high heat and fry the chicken breasts for about 3 minutes per side.

The chicken breasts must be transferred onto a paper towel-lined plate to drain.

At the bottom of a casserole, place about 1/2 cup of tomato sauce and spread evenly.

Arrange the chicken breasts over marinara sauce in a single layer.

Put sauce on top plus the mozzarella cheese slices.

Bake for about 20 minutes or until done completely.

Remove from the oven and serve hot with the garnishing of parsley.

Nutrition: Calories: 398 Fat: 15.1g Fiber: 9.4g Carbohydrates:4.1g Protein: 15.1g

62. CHICKEN ROLLATINI

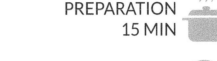

PREPARATION
15 MIN

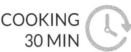

COOKING
30 MIN

SERVES
4

INGREDIENTS

- 4 (3-ounce) boneless skinless chicken breasts, pounded to about 1/3 inch thick
- 4 ounces ricotta cheese
- 4 slices prosciutto (4 ounces)
- 1 cup fresh spinach
- 1/2 cup almond flour
- 1/2 cup grated Parmesan cheese
- 2 eggs, beaten
- 1/4 cup good-quality olive oil

DIRECTIONS

Preheat the oven. Set the oven temperature to 400°F.

Prepare the chicken—Pat the chicken breasts dry with paper towels. Spread 1/4 of the ricotta in the middle of each breast.

Place the prosciutto over the ricotta and 1/4 cup of the spinach on the prosciutto.

Fold the long edges of the chicken breast over the filling, then roll the chicken breast up to enclose the filling.

Place the rolls seam-side down on your work surface.

Bread the chicken. On a plate, stir together the almond flour and Parmesan and set it next to the beaten eggs.

Carefully dip a chicken roll in the egg,

then roll it in the almond-flour mixture until it is completely covered.

Set the rolls seam-side down on your work surface. Repeat with the other rolls.

Brown the rolls. In a medium skillet over medium heat, warm the olive oil.

Place the rolls seam-side down in the skillet and brown them on all sides, turning them carefully, about 10 minutes in total.

Transfer the rolls, seam-side down, to a 9-by-9-inch baking dish—Bake the chicken rolls for 25 minutes, or until they're cooked through.

Serve. Place one chicken roll on each of four plates and serve them immediately.

Nutrition: Calories: 365 Fat: 17.1g Fiber: 9.4g Carbohydrates:3.2 g Protein: 1.4g

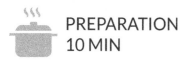

PREPARATION
10 MIN

COOKING
5 MIN

SERVES
2

63. LOW CARB BROCCOLI MASH

INGREDIENTS

▸ 325 g broccoli
▸ ½ clove garlic
▸ 2tablespoon parsley
▸ Salt
▸ 40 g butter
▸ Pepper

DIRECTIONS

Put salt into the water and boil. Put broccoli florets and cook within a few minutes. Remove the water and separate the soft broccoli.

Place all fixing in a blender and pulse. Serve.

Nutrition: Calories: 210 kcal Fats: 18 g Carbohydrates: 7 g Proteins: 5 g Fiber: 18 g

64. AVOCADO LOW CARB BURGER

PREPARATION
15 MIN
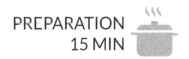

COOKING
25 MIN
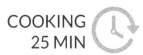

SERVES
4
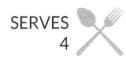

INGREDIENTS

- 1 avocado
- 1 leaf lettuce
- 2 slices of prosciutto or any ham
- 1 slice of tomato
- 1 egg
- ½ tbsp olive oil for frying
- **For the sauce:**
- 1 tbsp low carb mayonnaise
- ¼ tsp low carb hot sauce
- ¼ tsp mustard
- ¼ tsp Italian seasoning
- ½ tsp sesame seeds (optional

DIRECTIONS

In a small bowl, combine keto-friendly mayonnaise, mustard, hot sauce, and Italian seasoning

Heat 1/2 tablespoon of olive oil in a pan and cook an egg. The yolk must be fluid

Cut the avocado in half, remove the peel and bone. Cut the narrowest part of the avocado so that the fruit can stand on a plate

Fill the hole in one half of the avocado with the prepared sauce

Top with lettuce, prosciutto strips, a slice of tomato, and a fried egg

Cover with the other half of the avocado and sprinkle with sesame seeds (optional)

Nutrition: Calories: 416 kcal Carbs: 15 g Fat: 24 g Protein: 35 g

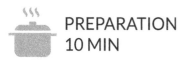

PREPARATION
10 MIN

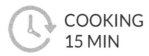

COOKING
15 MIN

SERVES
4

65. INCREDIBLE SALMON DISH

INGREDIENTS

- 3 cups of ice water
- 2 teaspoons sriracha sauce
- 4 teaspoons stevia
- 3 scallions, chopped
- Black pepper and salt to taste
- 2 teaspoons flaxseed oil
- 4 teaspoons apple cider vinegar
- 3 teaspoons avocado oil
- 4 medium salmon fillets
- 4 cups baby arugula

- 2 cups cabbage, finely chopped
- 1 and ½ teaspoon Jamaican jerk seasoning
- ¼ cup pepitas, toasted
- 2 cups watermelon radish, julienned

DIRECTIONS

Put ice water in a bowl, add scallions and leave aside.

In another bowl, mix sriracha sauce with stevia and stir well.

Transfer 2 teaspoons of this mix to a bowl and mix with half of the avocado oil, flaxseed oil, vinegar, salt and pepper, and whisk.

Sprinkle jerk seasoning over salmon, rub with sriracha and stevia mix and season with salt and pepper.

Heat-up a pan with the rest of the avocado oil over medium-high heat, add salmon, flesh side down, cook for 4 minutes, flip and cook for 4 minutes more and divide among plates.

In a bowl, mix radishes with cabbage and arugula.

Add salt, pepper, sriracha and vinegar mix and toss well.

Add this to salmon fillets, drizzle the remaining sriracha and stevia sauce all over and top with pepitas and drained scallions.

Enjoy!

Nutrition: Calories 160 kcal Fat 6g Fiber 1g Carbs 1g Protein 12g

PREPARATION
15 MIN

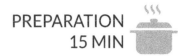

COOKING
15 MIN

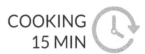

SERVES
2

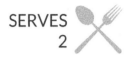

66. TANGY SHRIMP

INGREDIENTS

- ▶ Garlic (3)
- ▶ Olive oil (.25 cup)
- ▶ Jumbo shrimp (.5 lb.)
- ▶ Lemon (1)
- ▶ Cayenne pepper

DIRECTIONS

Sauté the garlic and cayenne with the olive oil.

 Peel and devein the shrimp.

Cook within 2 to 3 minutes per side.

Put pepper, salt, and lemon wedges.

Use the rest of the garlic oil for a dipping sauce. Serve.

Nutrition: Net Carbohydrates: 3 g Protein: 23 g Total Fats: 27 g Calories: 335 kcal

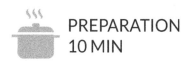

PREPARATION
10 MIN

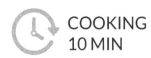

COOKING
10 MIN

SERVES
2

67. SCALLOPS AND FENNEL SAUCE

INGREDIENTS

- 6 scallops
- 1 fennel, trimmed, leaves chopped and bulbs cut in wedges
- Juice from ½ lime
- 1 lime, cut in wedges
- Zest from 1 lime
- 1 egg yolk
- 3 tablespoons ghee, melted and heated up
- ½ tablespoons olive oil
- Black pepper and salt to the taste

DIRECTIONS

Season scallops with salt and pepper, put in a bowl and mix with half of the lime juice and half of the zest and toss to coat.

In a bowl, mix the egg yolk with some salt and pepper, the rest of the lime juice and the rest of the lime zest and whisk well.

Add melted ghee and stir very well. Also, add fennel leaves and stir.

Brush fennel wedges with oil, place on heated grill over medium-high heat, cook for 2 minutes, flip and cook for 2 minutes more.

Add scallops on the grill, cook for 2 minutes, flip and cook for 2 minutes more.

Divide fennel and scallops on plates, drizzle fennel and ghee mix and serve with lime wedges on the side. Enjoy!

Nutrition: Calories 400 kcal Fat 24g Fiber 4g Carbs 12g Protein 25g

PREPARATION
10 MIN

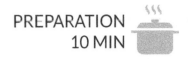

COOKING
1 H

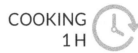

SERVES
2

68. SALMON AND LEMON RELISH

INGREDIENTS

- 2 medium salmon fillets
- Black pepper and salt to taste
- A drizzle of olive oil
- 1 shallot, chopped
- 1 tablespoon lemon juice
- 1 big lemon
- ¼ cup olive oil
- 2 tablespoons parsley, finely chopped

DIRECTIONS

Grease salmon fillets with olive oil, put salt and pepper, place on a lined baking sheet, standing in the oven at 400 °F, and bake for 1 hour

Stir 1 tablespoon lemon juice, salt, and pepper in a bowl and leave aside for 10 minutes

Cut the whole lemon in wedges and then very thinly

Put this in shallots, parsley, ¼ cup olive oil, and stir

Break the salmon into medium pieces and serve with the lemon relish on the side

Nutrition: Calories: 200 kcal Fat: 10 g Fiber: 1 g Carbs: 5 g Protein: 20 g

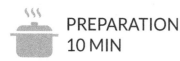

PREPARATION
10 MIN

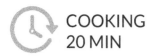

COOKING
20 MIN

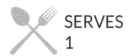

SERVES
1

69. MUSTARD GLAZED SALMON

INGREDIENTS

- ▶ 1 big salmon fillet
- ▶ Black pepper and salt to taste
- ▶ 2 tablespoons mustard
- ▶ 1 tablespoon coconut oil
- ▶ 1 tablespoon maple extract

DIRECTIONS

Mix maple extract with mustard in a bowl

Massage salmon with salt and pepper and half of the mustard mix

Heat-up a pan to high heat, place salmon flesh side down and cook for 5 minutes

Rub salmon with the rest of the mixture, transfer to a baking dish, place in the oven at 425 degrees F and bake for 15 minutes

Serve with a tasty side salad

Enjoy!

Nutrition: Calories 240 kcal Fat: 7 g Fiber: 1 g Carbs: 5 g Protein: 23

70. THAI PEANUT CHICKEN SKEWERS

PREPARATION
10 MIN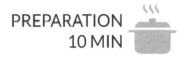

COOKING
15 MIN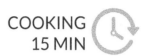

SERVES
2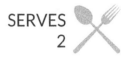

INGREDIENTS

- 1-pound boneless skinless chicken breast, cut into chunks
- 3 tablespoons coconut aminos
- 1/2 teaspoon Sriracha sauce, plus 1/4 teaspoon
- 3 teaspoons toasted sesame oil, divided
- Ghee, for oiling
- 2 tablespoons peanut butter
- Pink Himalayan salt
- Freshly ground black pepper

DIRECTIONS

In a bowl, combine the chicken chunks with two tablespoons of soy sauce, 1/2 teaspoon of Sriracha sauce, and two teaspoons of sesame oil. Marinate the chicken.

If you are using wood 8-inch skewers, soak them in water for 30 minutes before using.

Oil the grill pan with ghee.

Thread the chicken chunks onto the skewers.

Cook the skewers over low heat for 10 to 15 minutes, flipping halfway through.

Meanwhile, mix the peanut dipping sauce.

Stir together the remaining one tablespoon of soy sauce, 1/4 teaspoon of Sriracha sauce, one teaspoon of sesame oil, and the peanut butter.

Season with pink Himalayan salt and pepper.

Serve the chicken skewers with a small dish of the peanut sauce.

Nutrition: Calories: 390 Fat:18.4 g Fiber: 12.9g Carbohydrates:2.1 g Protein: 17.4g

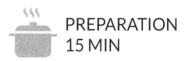

PREPARATION
15 MIN

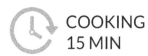

COOKING
15 MIN

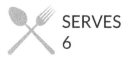

SERVES
6

71. TUSCAN CHICKEN

INGREDIENTS

- 11/2 pounds chicken breasts, pasteurized, skinless, thinly sliced
- 1/2 cup sun-dried tomatoes
- 1 cup spinach, chopped
- 1 teaspoon garlic powder
- 1 teaspoon Italian seasoning
- 2 tablespoons avocado oil
- 1/2 cup grated parmesan cheese
- 1 cup heavy cream, full-fat
- 1/2 cup chicken broth, pasteurized

DIRECTIONS

Take a large skillet pan, place it over medium-high heat, add oil, and when hot, add chicken and then cook for 3–5 minutes per side until golden brown.

Add garlic powder, Italian seasoning, and cheese into the pan, pour in the broth and cream, and then whisk until combined.

Switch heat to medium-high, cook the sauce for 2 minutes until it begins to thicken, then add tomatoes and spinach and simmer until spinach leaves begin to wilt.

Return chicken to the pan, toss until mixed, and cook for 2 minutes until hot.

Serve chicken with cooked Keto pasta, such as zucchini noodles.

Nutrition: Calories: 390 kcal Fat: 16.1g Fiber: 12.8g Carbohydrates: 3g Protein: 19g

72. LEMON BUTTER SAUCE WITH FISH

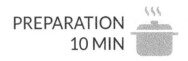

PREPARATION
10 MIN

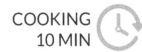

COOKING
10 MIN

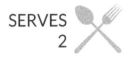

SERVES
2

INGREDIENTS

- 150 g thin white fish fillets
- 4 tbsp butter
- 2 tbsp white flour
- 2 tbsp olive oil
- 1 tbsp fresh lemon juice
- salt and pepper
- chopped parsley

DIRECTIONS

Place the butter in a small skillet over medium heat. Melt it and leave it, just stirring it casually.

After 3 mins, pour into a small bowl

Add lemon juice, season it, and set it aside

Dry the fish with paper towels, season it to taste, and sprinkle with flour

Heat oil in a skillet over high heat: when shimmering, add the fish and cook around 2-3 mins

Remove to a plate and serve with the sauce.

Top with parsley

Nutrition: Calories: 371 kcal Fats: 27 g Carbs: 3 g Protein: 30 g

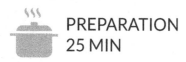

PREPARATION
25 MIN

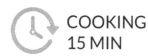

COOKING
15 MIN

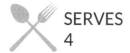

SERVES
4

73. COCONUT AND LIME STEAK

INGREDIENTS

- ▸ 2 pounds steak, grass-fed
- ▸ 1 tablespoon minced garlic
- ▸ 1 lime, zested
- ▸ 1 teaspoon ginger, grated
- ▸ 3/4 teaspoon sea salt
- ▸ 1 teaspoon red pepper flakes
- ▸ 2 tablespoons lime juice
- ▸ 1/2 cup coconut oil, melted

DIRECTIONS

Take a large bowl and add garlic, ginger, salt, red pepper flakes, lime juice, zest, pour in oil, and whisk until combined.

Add the steaks, toss until well coated, and marinate at room temperature for 20 minutes.

After 20 minutes, take a large skillet pan, place it over medium-high heat, and when hot, add steaks (cut steaks in half if they don't fit into the pan).

Cook the steaks and then transfer them to a cutting board.

Let steaks cool for 5 minutes, then slice across the grain and serve.

Nutrition: Calories: 512 Fat: 17.9g Fiber: 12.5g Carbohydrates:4.9 g Protein: 19.9g

74. BACON BLUE CHEESE FILLED EGGS

PREPARATION
10 MIN
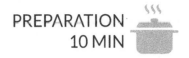

COOKING
90-120 MIN
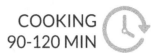

SERVES
3

INGREDIENTS

- 8 eggs
- ¼ cup crumbled blue cheese
- 3 slices of cooked bacon
- ¼ cup sour cream
- 1/3 cup mayo
- ¼ tsp pepper and dill
- ½ tsp salt
- 1 tbsp mustard
- parsley

DIRECTIONS

Hard boil your eggs and then cut them half. Place the yolks in a bowl

With a fork, mash the yolks, add the sour cream, mayo, bleu cheese, mustard, the seasoning, and mix until creamy enough for your taste.

Slice up the bacon to small pieces.

Stir in the rest of the Ingredients: and fill up the eggs.

Nutrition: Calories: 217 kcal Fats: 16 g Carbs: 1 g Protein: 6 g

PREPARATION
15 MIN

COOKING
5 MIN

SERVES
2

75. CHICKEN QUESADILLA

INGREDIENTS

- 1 tablespoon olive oil
- 2 low-carbohydrate tortillas
- ½ cup shredded Mexican blend cheese
- 2 ounces shredded chicken
- 2 tablespoons sour cream

DIRECTIONS

Warm-up, the olive oil in a large skillet, then put a tortilla, then top with ¼ cup of cheese, the chicken, the Tajin seasoning, and the remaining ¼ cup of cheese

Top with the second tortilla

Once the bottom tortilla gets golden, and the cheese begins to melt, after about 2 minutes, flip the quesadilla over

The second side will cook faster, about 1 minute

Once the second tortilla is crispy and golden, transfer the quesadilla to a cutting board and let sit for 2 minutes

Cut the quesadilla into 4 wedges using a pizza cutter or chef's knife

Transfer half the quesadilla to each of two plates

Put 1 tablespoon of sour cream and serve hot

Nutrition: Calories: 414 kcal Carbs: 24 g Protein: 26 g Fats: 28 g

76. SLOW COOKER BARBECUE RIBS

PREPARATION
15 MIN
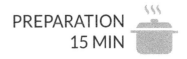

COOKING
4 H
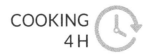

SERVES
2
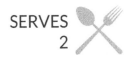

INGREDIENTS

- 1lb pork ribs
- Pink salt
- Freshly ground black pepper
- 1.25 oz package dry rib-seasoning rub
- ½ cup sugar-free barbecue sauce

DIRECTIONS

With the crock insert in place, preheat your slow cooker to high

Generously season the pork ribs with pink salt, pepper, and dry rib-seasoning rub

Stand the ribs up along the walls of the slow-cooker insert, with the bonier side facing inward

Pour the barbecue sauce on both sides of the ribs, using just enough to coat

Cover, cook for 4 hours, and serve

Nutrition: Calories: 373 kcal Carbohydrates: 1.8 g Protein: 46.7 g Fat: 18.6 g Sugar: 0.4 g Sodium: 231 mg Fiber: 0.7 g

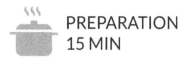

PREPARATION
15 MIN

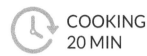

COOKING
20 MIN

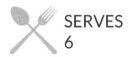

SERVES
6

77. HERBED GRILLED LAMB

INGREDIENTS

- 2 pounds of lamb
- 5 spoons of ghee butter
- 3 tablespoons of Keto mustard
- 2 minced garlic cloves
- 1 1/2 tablespoon of chopped basil
- 1/2 tablespoon of pepper
- 3 tablespoons of olive oil
- 1/2 teaspoon of salt

DIRECTIONS

Mix butter, mustard, and basil with a pinch of salt to taste. Then, set aside.

Mix garlic, salt, and pepper together. Then, add a teaspoon of oil.

Season the lamb generously with this mix.

Grill the lamb on medium heat until fully cooked.

Take butter mix and spread generously on chops and serve hot.

Nutrition: Calories: 390 kcal Fat: 19.5 g Fiber: 5.9g Carbohydrates: 3.2 g Protein: 18.6 g

78. BARBACOA BEEF ROAST

PREPARATION
15 MIN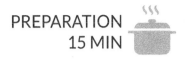

COOKING
8 H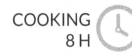

SERVES
4

INGREDIENTS

- ► 1 lb beef chuck roast
- ► 4 chipotle peppers in adobo sauce
- ► 6 oz can green jalapeño chilis
- ► 2 tablespoons apple cider vinegar
- ► ½ cup beef broth

DIRECTIONS

With the crock insert in place, preheat your slow cooker to low

Massage the beef chuck roast on both sides with pink salt and pepper

Put the roast in the slow cooker

Pulse the chipotle peppers and their adobo sauce, jalapeños, and apple cider vinegar in a blender

Add the beef broth and pulse a few more times

Pour the chili mixture over the top of the roast

Cover and cook on low within 8 hours, then shred the meat and serve hot

Nutrition: Calories: 723 kcal Carbs: 7 g Protein: 66 g Fats: 46 g

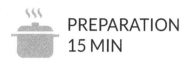

PREPARATION
15 MIN

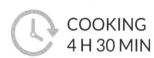

COOKING
4 H 30 MIN

SERVES
2

79. BEEF & BROCCOLI ROAST

INGREDIENTS

- 1 lb. beef chuck roast
- ½ cup beef broth
- Soy sauce, ¼ cup
- 1 teaspoon toasted sesame oil
- 1 (16-ounce) bag frozen broccoli

DIRECTIONS

With the crock insert in place, preheat your slow cooker to low

On a cutting board, season the chuck roast with pink salt, pepper, and slice the roast thin

Put the sliced beef in your slow cooker

Combine sesame oil and beef broth in a small bowl then pour over the beef

Cover and cook on low for 4 hours

Add the frozen broccoli and cook for 30 minutes more

If you need more liquid, add additional beef broth. Serve hot

Nutrition: Calories: 803 kcal Carbs: 18 g Protein: 74 g Fats: 49 g

80. LOADED CAULIFLOWER SALAD

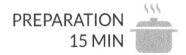

PREPARATION
15 MIN

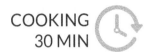

COOKING
30 MIN

SERVES
4

INGREDIENTS

- ▸ One large head cauliflower
- ▸ Six slices bacon
- ▸ 1/2 c. sour cream
- ▸ 1/4 c. mayonnaise
- ▸ 1 tbsp. lemon juice
- ▸ 1/2 tsp. garlic powder
- ▸ Kosher salt
- ▸ ground black pepper
- ▸ 1 1/2 c. cheddar
- ▸ 1/4 c. chives

DIRECTIONS

Boil 1/4 water, put cauliflower, cover pan and steam within 4 minutes. Drain and cool.

Cook the pork around 3 minutes per side. Drain then cut.

Mix the sour cream, mayonnaise, lemon juice, and garlic powder in a big bowl. Toss the cauliflower florets. Put salt pepper, bacon, cheddar, and chives. Serve.

Nutrition: Calories 440 kcal Protein 19 g Carbohydrates 13 g Fiber 4 g Fat 35 g

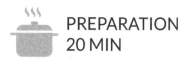

PREPARATION
20 MIN

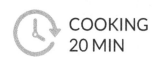

COOKING
20 MIN

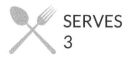

SERVES
3

81. PESTO PORK CHOPS

INGREDIENTS

▸ 3 (3-ounce) top-flood pork chops, boneless, fat
▸ 8 tablespoons Herb Pesto (here)
▸ ½ cup bread crumbs
▸ 1 tablespoon olive oil

DIRECTIONS

Preheat the oven to 360 ° F

Cover a foil baker's sheet; set aside

Rub 1 tablespoon of pesto evenly across each pork chop on both sides

Every pork chop in the crumbs of bread is lightly dredged

Heat the oil in a medium-high heat large skillet

Brown the pork chops for about 6 minutes on each side

Place on the baking sheet the pork chops

Bake until the pork reaches 136 °F in the center for about 10 minutes

Nutrition: Fat: 8 g Carbohydrates: 10 g Phosphorus: 188 mg Potassium: 220 mg Sodium: 138 mg Protein: 23 g Calories 815 kcal

82. SALMON PASTA

PREPARATION
15 MIN
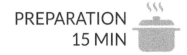

COOKING
1 H 30 MIN
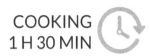

SERVES
2
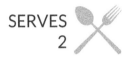

INGREDIENTS

- Coconut oil (2 tbsp.)
- Zucchinis (2)
- Smoked salmon (8 oz.)
- Keto-friendly mayo (.25 cup)

DIRECTIONS

Make noodle-like strands from the zucchini.

Warm-up, the oil, put the salmon and sauté within 2 to 3 minutes.

Stir in the noodles and sauté for 1 to 2 more minutes.

Stir in the mayo and serve.

Nutrition: Net Carbohydrates: 3 g Protein: 21 g Total Fats: 42 g Calories: 470 kcal

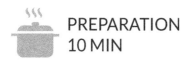

PREPARATION
10 MIN

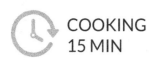

COOKING
15 MIN

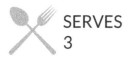

SERVES
3

83. ASPARAGUS SALAD

INGREDIENTS

- 10 oz asparagus
- 1 tablespoon olive oil
- ½ teaspoon white pepper
- 4 oz Feta cheese, crumbled
- 1 cup lettuce, chopped
- 1 tablespoon canola oil
- 1 teaspoon apple cider vinegar
- 1 tomato, diced

DIRECTIONS

Preheat the oven to 365 °F

Place asparagus in the tray, sprinkle with olive oil, white pepper, and transfer to the preheated oven. Cook it for 15 minutes

Meanwhile, put crumbled Feta in the salad bowl

Add chopped lettuce and diced tomato

Sprinkle the ingredients with apple cider vinegar

Chill the cooked asparagus to room temperature and add in the salad

Shake the salad gently before serving

Nutrition: Calories: 87.5 kcal Total Fat: 4.1 g Cholesterol: 9.2 mg Sodium: 685.8 mg Potassium: 212.1 mg Total Carbohydrate: 8.1 g Protein: 5.1 g

PREPARATION
5 MIN
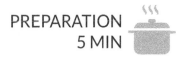

COOKING
18 MIN
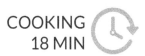

SERVES
2
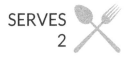

84. BEEF WITH CABBAGE NOODLES

INGREDIENTS

- 4 oz ground beef
- 1 cup chopped cabbage
- 4 oz tomato sauce
- ½ tsp minced garlic
- ½ cup of water
- **Seasoning:**
- ½ tbsp coconut oil
- ½ tsp salt
- ¼ tsp Italian seasoning
- 1/8 tsp dried basil

DIRECTIONS

Take a skillet pan, place it over medium heat, add oil and when hot, add beef and cook for 5 minutes until nicely browned

Meanwhile, prepare the cabbage and, for it, slice the cabbage into thin shred

When the beef has cooked, add garlic, season with salt, basil, and Italian seasoning, stir well and continue cooking for 3 minutes until beef has thoroughly cooked

Pour in tomato sauce and water, stir well and bring the mixture to boil

Then reduce heat to medium-low level, add cabbage, stir well until well mixed and simmer for 3 to 5 minutes until cabbage is softened, covering the pan

Uncover the pan and continue simmering the beef until most of the cooking liquid has evaporated

Serve

Nutrition: Calories: 188.5 kcal Fats: 12.5 g Protein: 15.5 g Net Carbohydrates: 2.5 g Fiber: 1 g

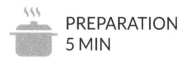

PREPARATION
5 MIN

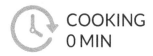

COOKING
0 MIN

SERVES
2

85. ROAST BEEF AND MOZZARELLA PLATE

INGREDIENTS

- ► 4 slices of roast beef
- ► ½ ounce chopped lettuce
- ► 1 avocado, pitted
- ► 2 oz mozzarella cheese, cubed
- ► ½ cup mayonnaise
- ► **Seasoning:**
- ► ¼ tsp salt
- ► 1/8 tsp ground black pepper
- ► 2 tbsp avocado oil

DIRECTIONS

Scoop out flesh from avocado and divide it evenly between two plates

Add slices of roast beef, lettuce, cheese, and then sprinkle with salt and black pepper

Serve with avocado oil and mayonnaise

Nutrition: Calories: 267.7 kcal Fats: 24.5 g Protein: 9.5 g Net Carbohydrates: 1.5 g Fiber: 2 g

PREPARATION
5 MIN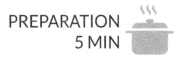

COOKING
10 MIN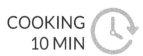

SERVES
2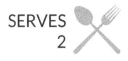

86. BEEF AND BROCCOLI

INGREDIENTS

- ▶ 6 slices of beef roast, cut into strips
- ▶ 1 scallion, chopped
- ▶ 3 oz broccoli florets, chopped
- ▶ 1 tbsp avocado oil
- ▶ 1 tbsp butter, unsalted
- ▶ **Seasoning:**
- ▶ ¼ tsp salt
- ▶ 1/8 tsp ground black pepper
- ▶ 1 ½ tbsp soy sauce
- ▶ 3 tbsp chicken broth

DIRECTIONS

Take a medium skillet pan, place it over medium heat, add oil and when hot, add beef strips and cook for 2 minutes until hot

Transfer beef to a plate, add scallion to the pan, then add butter and cook for 3 minutes until tender

Add remaining ingredients, stir until mixed, switch heat to the low level, and simmer for 3 to 4 minutes until broccoli is tender

Return beef to the pan, stir until well combined, and cook for 1 minute.

Serve

Nutrition: Calories: 15.7 kcal Fats: 21.6 g Protein: 1.7 g Net Carbohydrates:1.3 g

PREPARATION
5 MIN

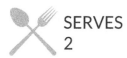 **COOKING**
10 MIN

SERVES
2

87. GARLIC HERB BEEF ROAST

INGREDIENTS

- ▸ 6 slices of beef roast
- ▸ ½ tsp garlic powder
- ▸ 1/3 tsp dried thyme
- ▸ ¼ tsp dried rosemary
- ▸ 2 tbsp butter, unsalted
- ▸ **Seasoning:**
- ▸ 1/3 tsp salt
- ▸ 1/4 tsp ground black pepper

DIRECTIONS

Prepare the spice mix and for this, take a small bowl, place garlic powder, thyme, rosemary, salt, black pepper and then stir until mixed

Sprinkle spice mix on the beef roast

Take a medium skillet pan, place it over medium heat, add butter and when it melts, add beef roast and then cook for 5 to 8 minutes until golden brown and cooked

Serve

Nutrition: Calories: 140 kcal Fats: 12.7 g Protein: 5.5 g Net Carbohydrates: 0.1 g Fiber: 0.2 g

88. SPROUTS STIR-FRY WITH KALE, BROCCOLI, AND BEEF

PREPARATION
5 MIN
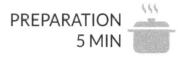

COOKING
8 MIN
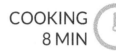

SERVES
2
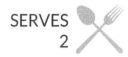

INGREDIENTS

- 3 slices of beef roast, chopped
- 2 oz Brussels sprouts, halved
- 4 oz broccoli florets
- 3 oz kale
- 1 ½ tbsp butter, unsalted
- 1/8 tsp red pepper flakes
- **Seasoning:**
- ¼ tsp garlic powder
- ¼ tsp salt
- 1/8 tsp ground black pepper

DIRECTIONS

Take a medium skillet pan, place it over medium heat, add ¾ tbsp butter and when it melts, add broccoli florets, sprouts, sprinkle with garlic powder, and cook for 2 minutes

Season vegetables with salt and red pepper flakes, add chopped beef, stir until mixed and continue cooking for 3 minutes until browned on one side

Then add kale along with remaining butter, flip the vegetables and cook for 2 minutes until kale leaves wilts

Serve

Nutrition: Calories: 125 kcal Fats: 9.4 g Protein: 4.8 g Net Carbohydrates: 1.7 g Fiber: 2.6 g

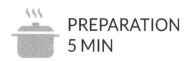

PREPARATION
5 MIN

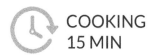

COOKING
15 MIN

SERVES
2

89. BEEF AND VEGETABLE SKILLET

INGREDIENTS

- ▶ 3 oz spinach, chopped
- ▶ ½ pound ground beef
- ▶ 2 slices of bacon, diced
- ▶ 2 oz chopped asparagus
- ▶ **Seasoning:**
- ▶ 3 tbsp coconut oil
- ▶ 2 tsp dried thyme
- ▶ 2/3 tsp salt
- ▶ ½ tsp ground black pepper

DIRECTIONS

Take a skillet pan, place it over medium heat, add oil and when hot, add beef and bacon and cook for 5 to 7 minutes until slightly browned

Then add asparagus and spinach, sprinkle with thyme, stir well and cook for 7 to 10 minutes until thoroughly cooked

Season skillet with salt and black pepper and serve

Nutrition: Calories: 332.5 kcal Fats: 26 g Protein : 23.5 g Carbohydrates: 1.5 g Fiber: 1 g

90. BEEF, PEPPER AND GREEN BEANS STIR-FRY

PREPARATION
5 MIN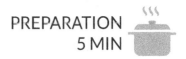

COOKING
18 MIN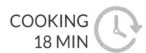

SERVES
2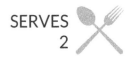

INGREDIENTS

- ▶ 6 oz ground beef
- ▶ 2 oz chopped green bell pepper
- ▶ 4 oz green beans
- ▶ 3 tbsp grated cheddar cheese
- ▶ **Seasoning:**
- ▶ ½ tsp salt
- ▶ ¼ tsp ground black pepper
- ▶ ¼ tsp paprika

. . . .

DIRECTIONS

Take a skillet pan, place it over medium heat, add ground beef and cook for 4 minutes until slightly browned

Then add bell pepper, green beans, season with salt, paprika, black pepper, stir well and continue cooking for 7 to 10 minutes until beef and vegetables have cooked through

Sprinkle cheddar cheese on top, then transfer pan under the broiler and cook for 2 minutes until cheese has melted and the top is golden brown

Serve

Nutrition: Calories: 282.5 kcal Fats: 17.6 g Protein: 26.1 g Net Carbohydrates: 2.9 g

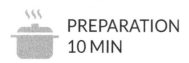

PREPARATION
10 MIN

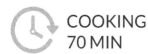

COOKING
70 MIN

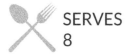

SERVES
8

91. ROASTED PORK LOIN WITH BROWN MUSTARD SAUCE

INGREDIENTS

- 1 (2-pound) boneless pork loin roast
- Sea salt
- Freshly ground black pepper
- 3 tablespoons olive oil
- 11/2 cups heavy (whipping) cream
- 3 tablespoons grainy mustard, such as Pommery

DIRECTIONS

Preheat the oven to 375°F.

Season the pork roast all over with sea salt and pepper.

Heat oil then all the sides of the roast must be browned, about 6 minutes in total, and place the roast in a baking dish.

When there are approximately 15 minutes of roasting time left, place a small saucepan over medium heat and add the heavy cream and mustard.

Stir the sauce until it simmers, then reduce the heat to low. Simmer the sauce until it is vibrant and thick, about 5 minutes. Remove the pan from the heat and set aside.

Nutrition: Calories: 415 kcal Fat: 18.4g Fiber: 11.3g Carbohydrates:3.1 g Protein: 17.4g

CHAPTER 9: 30 DAY MEAL PLAN

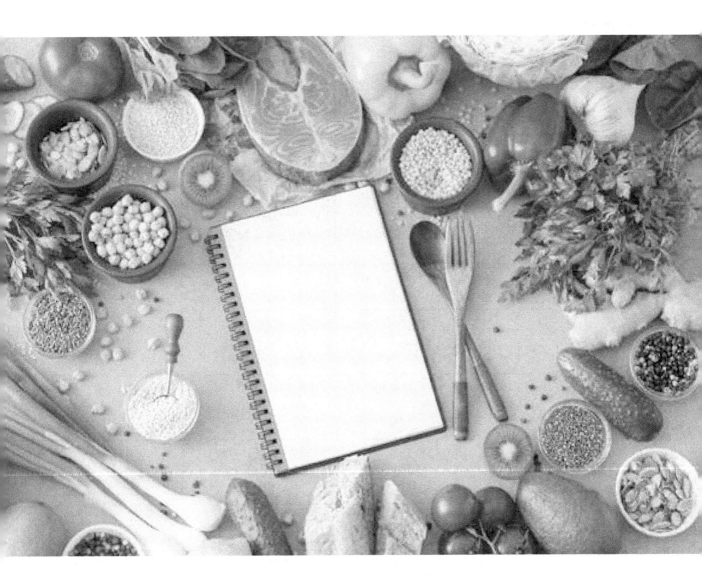

DAY	BREAKFAST	LUNCH	DINNER
1	YOGURT WAFFLES	MUSHROOM & CAULIFLOWER RISOTTO	CHICKEN QUESADILLA
2	BROCCOLI MUFFINS	PITA PIZZA	BEEF AND BROCCOLI
3	PUMPKIN BREAD	SPICY KETO CHICKEN WINGS	BACON BLUE CHEESE FILLED EGGS
4	SPINACH ARTICHOKE BREAKFAST BAKE	TACO CASSEROLE	KORMA CURRY
5	GRANOLA BARS	STICKY PORK RIBS	CHICKEN PARMIGIANA
6	GINGER FRENCH TOAST	KETO CROQUE MONSIEUR	TANGY SHRIMP
7	BAGELS WITH CHEESE	KETO WRAPS WITH CREAM CHEESE AND SALMON	STUFFED PORTOBELLO MUSHROOMS
8	BAKED APPLES	BEEF WELLINGTON	PESTO FLAVORED STEAK
9	OMELET WITH PEPPERS	BROCCOLI AND CHICKEN CASSEROLE	FLAWLESS GRILLED STEAK
10	GINGER FRENCH TOAST	CREAMY SCALLOPS	BRUSSELS SPROUTS WITH BACON
11	YOGURT WAFFLES	PERFECT PAN-SEARED SCALLOPS	CREAMY ZOODLES
12	BROCCOLI MUFFINS	EASY BAKED SHRIMP SCAMPI	COFFEE BBQ PORK BELLY
13	PUMPKIN BREAD	DELICIOUS BLACKENED SHRIMP	GARLIC & THYME LAMB CHOPS

14	SPINACH ARTICHOKE BREAKFAST BAKE	SIGNATURE ITALIAN PORK DISH	JAMAICAN JERK PORK ROAST
15	GRANOLA BARS	FLAVOR PACKED PORK LOIN	KETO MEATBALLS
16	GINGER FRENCH TOAST	SPICED PORK TENDERLOIN	MIXED VEGETABLE PATTIES - INSTANT POT
17	BAGELS WITH CHEESE	STICKY PORK RIBS	ROASTED LEG OF LAMB
18	BAKED APPLES	LOW-CALORIE CHEESY BROCCOLI QUICHE	MONGOLIAN BEEF
19	OMELET WITH PEPPERS	LOW CARB BROCCOLI LEEK SOUP	LETTUCE SALAD
20	AVOCADO EGG BOWLS	ITALIAN STYLE HALIBUT PACKETS	GRAIN-FREE CREAMY NOODLES
21	YOGURT WAFFLES	SPICY KETO CHICKEN WINGS	MEAT-FREE ZOODLES STROGANOFF
22	BROCCOLI MUFFINS	CHEESY HAM QUICHE	EYE-CATCHING VEGGIES
23	PUMPKIN BREAD	BROCCOLI AND CHICKEN CASSEROLE	SALMON AND LEMON RELISH
24	SPINACH ARTICHOKE BREAKFAST BAKE	LAMB CHOPS AND HERB BUTTER	CHICKEN PARMIGIANA
25	GRANOLA BARS	BEEF WELLINGTON	CREAMY ZOODLES

26	GINGER FRENCH TOAST	BUTTERED COD	BACON BLUE CHEESE FILLED EGGS
27	BAGELS WITH CHEESE	SALMON WITH RED CURRY SAUCE	PESTO PORK CHOPS
28	BAKED APPLES	SALMON TERIYAKI	BEEF WITH CABBAGE NOODLES
29	OMELET WITH PEPPERS	ITALIAN STYLE HALIBUT PACKETS	BEEF, PEPPER AND GREEN BEANS STIR-FRY
30	AVOCADO EGG BOWLS	CHICKEN CASSEROLE	TANGY SHRIMP

CONCLUSION

The ketogenic diet is one that has many important aspects and information that you need to know as someone who wants to try this diet. It is important to remember the warning that we have given you at the beginning of the book that this is not a diet that is safe and that doctors recommend you don't try it, or if you are going to attempt it remember that you shouldn't do so for longer than six months and even then never without the constant supervision of a doctor or at the very least a doctor knowing that you're doing this and you following their guidelines and words exactly so that they can make sure that you are safe.

The ketogenic diet is a diet that believes that by minimizing your carbs, you will while maximizing the good fat in your system and making sure that you're getting the protein you need, that you will be happier and healthier. In this book, we give you the information to know what this diet is all about, as well as describing the different types and areas that this diet will offer. Most people assume that there is only one way to do this, and while there is one thing that the additional options share, there are actually four different options you can choose from. Each one has it's unique benefits, and you should know about each type to learn what would be best for your body, which is why we have described them in the book for you to have the best information possible when you begin this diet for yourself.

Another big thing about this diet is that many people don't understand the importance of exercise with this diet. The best way to become healthier is to do three things for yourself. Get the right amount of sleep, eat healthily, and make sure that you get the proper amount of exercise as well for your body to work at an optimum level. As such, we explain the exercises that are the best to go with your diet to make sure that you are getting the most out of it.

For women who are on the go and have a busy lifestyle, we have provided recipes for a thirty-day meal plan so that you can make food quickly and have a great meal for your lifestyle. They also have enough servings for you to have leftovers so that you don't have to worry about preparing in the morning. Instead, you can simply pack it up and take it with you wherever you go. This works out so much easier for so many people because they don't have to cook in the morning, and it saves a busy person a lot of time.

We also provide helpful ideas on how you can use these recipes for meals to make sure that you see how the numbers will affect you and make an impact on your day. A great example that we have explained is if you have a big breakfast that is full of the protein you need, for example, thirty g, you've got to take note of this and be aware because if you eat too much for your dinner or another meal, you will throw your numbers out of where they are supposed to be. For those that have more time on their hands, we offer a thirty-day meal plan for you as well with all-new recipes to enjoy and tips and tricks for making them work for you in the best way.

With all of this information at your fingertips, you will be able to enjoy this diet and use it to your advantage. Another benefit that we offer? We explain routines that you can do for yourself to make this diet last longer for you and to benefit your body better as a result. Routines are very important and can be a big help to your body but also your spirit and your mind. This will help you utilize the diet better, and you will be able to improve with it as well as have it become easier for you to handle.

As many people are using this diet to their benefit, knowing your food is one of the biggest parts of this, and it becomes easier once you begin to use this in your daily life. One of the best things you can do is pay attention to the food that you are eating and how it affects your body and mind. You will notice that this diet has the ability to make you sick, which isn't a good thing, and it's one of the things the doctors warn against. For this reason, it's very important to pay attention to what you are eating and how your feeling at the same time. Another warning that we have said you need to pay attention to is that you will need to make sure that your ketogenic 'flu' isn't the result of something more serious. As people are being told that this is normal, this book has brought you the knowledge you need to be able to tell you why it's not.

This book has given you all the information you need to do this diet properly and to do it well. It's important to understand what you're getting into when you go into this diet, and this book will give you valuable information that you can use to your benefit and so you can avoid the problems that can come with this diet. You want to stay healthy and make sure that your body is able to do what it needs to. As with anything, we have put a strong emphasis on the fact that if anything feels wrong or unnatural, you will need to see a doctor to make sure that you are safe and that your body can handle this diet. Use the knowledge in this book to have amazing recipes and learn directions for amazing meals for yourself.

CPSIA information can be obtained
at www.ICGtesting.com
Printed in the USA
LVHW060019220221
679574LV00006B/367